WOMEN'S EXPERIENCE
OF FEMINIST THERAPY
AND COUNSELLING

WOMEN'S EXPERIENCE OF FEMINIST THERAPY AND COUNSELLING

Eileen McLeod

OPEN UNIVERSITY PRESS
Buckingham · Philadelphia

Open University Press
Celtic Court
22 Ballmoor
Buckingham
MK18 1XW

and

1900 Frost Road, Suite 101
Bristol, PA 19007, USA

First Published 1994

A catalogue record of this book is available from the British Library

ISBN 0–335–19222–X. – ISBN 0–335–19221–1 (pbk.)

Library of Congress Cataloging-in-Publication Data
McLeod, Eileen.
   Women's experience of feminist therapy and counselling / Eileen
McLeod
      p.   cm.
   Includes bibliographical references and index.
   ISBN 0–335–19222–X. – ISBN 0–335–19221–1 (pbk.)
   1. Feminist therapy. 2. Women – Mental health. 3. Patient
satisfaction. I. Title.
RC489.F45M38   1994
   616.89'14–dc20   93–40802
                                                              CIP

Typeset by Type Study, Scarborough
Printed in Great Britain by St Edmundsbury Press,
Bury St Edmunds, Suffolk

To Cleo
Born 4 June 1993

Contents

Acknowledgements

I would like to thank the University of Warwick for a grant from the Research and Innovations Fund, which funded the research on which this book is based.

I would like to acknowledge and thank Christina Hughes for her work as co-researcher, and Helen Evers for her assistance with initial analysis.

I would also like to thank Hilary Pugh who typed and retyped her way through the manuscript with the greatest skill. Louise Bellanti, Sonia Conmy, Marcie Edwards and Margaret Meredith, also carried out splendid work in typing additional materials.

I am very grateful to everyone who read the book in draft: David Howe, Pauline McManus, Julia Powell, Elaine Pullen, Lesley Stewart and Karen Stone.

I would also like to thank Heidi Sellwood whose excellent work freed up time, energy and concentration. Finally, I would like to thank Anna, my daughter, for her loving and brilliant contribution across the summer of Phoenix, Sitges and 'the Book'.

one

Emotional wellbeing for women: the development of feminist therapy and counselling

Introduction

This book analyses the significance for women's emotional wellbeing of their experience of feminist therapy and counselling. It springs from an observation, a discovery and a perception. The observation is that so many women are unhappy, despite being in relationships that are supposed to promote emotional wellbeing. The discovery is that feminist therapy and counselling can foster women's happiness. The perception is that so much more work needs to be done to realize women's happiness.

Feminist therapy and counselling is one of the elements in contemporary feminist action concerned with women's emotional wellbeing. The cornerstone of its development has been to locate the origins of widespread emotional suffering amongst women, in the gendered nature of social relations. As a mode of intervention, it has created forms of interaction in therapy, counselling, groupwork and resource centres aimed at more genuinely meeting women's emotional needs.

By now feminist therapy and counselling has grown to the point where there are centres of practice and networks of practitioners across the United States (Rosewater and Walker 1985; Burstow 1992), in other countries – for example Australia and New Zealand (see respectively Louisa Lawson Centre 1992; Wellington Eating Disorder Support 1992), and around Britain (Women in Mind 1986; Heenan 1988; Barnes and Maple 1992). Thousands of women have engaged in its activities as practitioners, beneficiaries and on a self-help basis. A substantial popular and scholarly literature has evolved (see respectively Ernst and Goodison 1981; Eichenbaum and Orbach 1984; and Brown and Liss-Levinson 1981; Brown 1990).

However, although the growth of feminist therapy and counselling indicates that it is sought after, it cannot be assumed to be benefiting women.

Major issues explored in this book

Making progress on understanding and evaluating the benefits of feminist therapy is hampered by the dearth of material from the viewpoint of women beneficiaries. This shortfall seems strange in a feminist initiative. Women relating their perceptions of their own experience, as opposed to assumptions being made about its positive nature, has been a major force in propelling feminist action into existence and in moving it on. The distinctive contribution of this book is that it does draw on the views of women beneficiaries of feminist therapy and counselling to assess its significance. This makes it possible to begin to understand what women actually find helpful and unhelpful about feminist therapy: for example, what lies behind the glowing endorsement from *Debbie*, one woman in our study:

> But considering how many times I came in hours and the impact that's had on my life, it's phenomenal. Thirty years of being on this earth and you feel you know yourself fairly well, then for it to be turned on its head, to be able to cope better, love more effectively. Those hours were golden, really.

The question of what women find unhelpful is also opened up, something which may be denied to therapists themselves. *Gillian*, in our study, said:

> I lied to her. I said 'Yes, I've solved my problems, I'm all right now.' But really I wasn't, because I kept thinking I was boring her. I didn't want to carry on any more. I let her believe I was cured.

Most existing accounts of feminist therapy and counselling have been written by therapists and counsellors themselves, whether handbooks for practitioners (e.g. Chaplin 1988; Burstow 1992); or generalized accounts of its aims and orientations (e.g. Eichenbaum and Orbach 1984, 1985; Walker 1990); or analyses and evaluations of practice (e.g. Ernst and Maguire 1987). Accounts of feminist therapy and counselling written by therapists and counsellors may be critical of their own work, and may use case examples drawn from actual experience (e.g. Lawrence 1984). Such examples are still being selected by the therapists and counsellors. They also tend to be treated as ideal types and written up in the therapists' and counsellors' words (e.g. Eichenbaum and Orbach 1984, 1985; Maguire 1987). At times they are created as ideal types as in Chaplin's account: 'The three clients, Julia, Mary and Louise, are actually fictional characters made up from a number of different clients, students and friends' (Chaplin 1988: 2). In the rare instances where case examples are offered in the beneficiaries' own words (e.g.

Woodward 1988) they still represent the therapist's selection from an unspecified population. Where autobiographical accounts exist (e.g. Spring 1987), they reflect an individual's experience.

None of these types of work meets the need for finding out independently the views of the significance of feminist therapy and counselling across a population of women coming to a centre of practice so that conclusions about its positive and negative effects can begin to be drawn. This study provides this through obtaining the views of a sample of the population of women who attended a provisional feminist therapy and counselling centre in Britain in its first two years of operation. The views of the counsellors and coordinator at the centre have also been obtained. (See Appendix 2 and Appendix 3 for profiles of the women participants and the counsellors and coordinator of the therapy and counselling centre.)

Three further major issues require attention when weighing the benefits of feminist therapy.

1 The limitations to analysing the state of women's emotional wellbeing solely in terms of subordination through gender.
2 How egalitarian are the theories therapists and counsellors employ and the activities they institute.
3 How egalitarian are the outcomes of feminist therapy and counselling.

These three major issues, explored through the views and experience of women participants and counsellors engaged in feminist therapy and counselling, form the nub of this book.

Structure of this book

The remainder of this chapter after the Introduction discusses each of these three issues in turn. Each is analysed in two ways:

● How the development of feminist therapy and counselling has raised it as an issue that needs to be explored when the contribution of feminist therapy and counselling to women's emotional wellbeing is being assessed.
● How this book explores the issue in question, together with the nature of the research.

The research for this book was designed and carried out with Christina Hughes as co-researcher. (Details of sampling and interviewing procedures are in Appendix 1.)

Chapters 2 and 3 then examine the first major issue: the limitations to analysing the state of women's emotional wellbeing, only in terms of subordination through gender. These limitations cannot be deduced solely from women participants' accounts of their experience during feminist therapy. Therefore, they are explored through the women's accounts of what they identify as primary personal relationships in childhood and adulthood, e.g. with parents and partners. Such relationships are revealed as arenas in which the interplay of a range of social inequalities has a profound impact on women's emotional wellbeing.

Chapter 4 then draws on the counsellors' and coordinators' accounts to review the second major issue: how egalitarian the theories' organization, procedures and activities instituted in the name of feminist therapy and counselling seem to be. This is gauged against the picture from the women's accounts of the way in which social inequalities informed their emotional wellbeing. The impact of the organization and practice of feminist therapy on the emotional wellbeing of its practitioners as workers is also examined.

Chapter 5, on the basis of women participants' accounts, explores the remaining major issue: how egalitarian are the outcomes of feminist therapy and counselling. Feminist therapy may be egalitarian in intent, but this does not guarantee that its outcomes are egalitarian. The reasons why women seek feminist therapy and counselling and the extent to which it promotes their emotional wellbeing through resolving the unequal social relations under-mining it are the lynchpins of analysis.

Finally, Chapter 6 specifies the combination of existing features in the theory, organization and practice of feminist therapy, together with further developments, which seem necessary if it is to contribute to a more equitable experience of emotional wellbeing.

Author's perspective

My interest in women's experience of feminist therapy and counselling stems from three sources. First, in my own experience and from that of women relatives and friends and from my previous research (Leonard and McLeod 1980; McLeod 1982; Dominelli and McLeod 1989; Chs 1 and 3), women's emotional wellbeing seems fraught, and the contribution of personal relationships which in theory should foster it problematic. Second, as a result of engaging in campaigning and social work from a feminist perspective, I am interested in how feminist initiatives fare in their attempts to create more egalitarian relationships, and in learning from the ensuing difficulties, what might be required to gain greater purchase on dissolving the social inequalities women face (McLeod 1982; Dominelli and McLeod 1989). Third, my interest developed as a result of contacting the feminist therapy and counselling centre featured in this book. I was allowed to read the anonymous follow-up returns of women who had been to the Centre. About 80 per cent of the women who had been counselled at the Centre had replied and were uniformly positive about what they had gained, contrasting this with their previous desperate state. This suggested that it would be important to analyse the practice of feminist therapy and counselling of which the Centre's work was an example.

I am conscious that what I write is mediated by my own social circumstances: I am a white, English, middle-class, 48-year-old, disabled, heterosexual woman, and a single parent. My understanding of other women's experience is bound to be partial; at the same time it is important to try to give an account of the need for women to have their emotional requirements met whatever their social circumstances.

Using the term 'women' in the title and discussion of this book in an unqualified way implies a view of women's experience as generic, disregarding differences between women. This is not my position. However, finding an alternative form of expression, which did not exclude the nature and nuances of other women's experience as equally important, proved impossible. What I have done, therefore, is to retain the term, but in the course of writing try to make the point that 'women's' experience is highly differentiated, and that only as feminist initiatives reflect this are they likely to be of benefit.

It is neither the purpose of this book, nor in its design, to tease out the possible organic origins of emotional distress as experienced by the women concerned. However, evidence exists that poor physical health is associated with emotional suffering (Smith and Jacobson 1989). Moreover, the impact of ill health and disability on emotional wellbeing stalks the women's accounts presented here. Therefore, the aim is to relate how women's own responses and those of others to ill health and disability reflect prevailing social inequalities, with consequences for their emotional wellbeing.

As discussed later in the chapter, some schools of thought within feminist therapy, drawing on the psychoanalytic tradition, have emphasized the importance of unconscious processes in shaping women's behaviour. However, this study does not seek to unravel what may be unconscious determinants of behaviour. Instead it confines itself to analysing the women's, the counsellors' and the coordinator's accounts, as the products of conscious thought.

Finally, it is beyond the remit of this book to focus on men's experience. However, it is not assumed that men's behaviour has uniformly negative effects on women (see Dominelli and McLeod 1989), nor that it is free from the damaging effects of unequal social relations. Instead, evidence is considered on the case for practice relating to men's emotional welfare being a valid feminist project.

Terminology

Anyone currently writing on feminist therapy faces the issue of whether or not the terms *feminist therapy/counselling* and *therapists/counsellors* should be used interchangeably (Walker 1990: x). This issue reflects the complexities of the aetiology of feminist therapy. It is further complicated by the term *counselling* being used in Britain, when in America the same activity might be referred to as therapy.

Some practitioners of feminist therapy have concentrated on trying to work out how psychotherapeutic insights and practices can be used or transformed from a feminist perspective, so that women's wellbeing is served (e.g. Eichenbaum and Orbach 1987). In this case referring to practice solely as feminist therapy, and to the practitioners as feminist therapists may seem appropriate.

However, there are several arguments for the interchangeability of the terms. First, women from backgrounds in both counselling and psychotherapy have gone on to develop a feminist perspective in their work and typified themselves as feminist therapists (Heenan 1988). Therefore they are likely to carry out practice which reflects both traditions. Second, as Mearns and Dryden argue, counselling and psychotherapy have features in common (although I would not agree with their assumption about what constitutes a 'deepseated' experience).

> Sometimes workers will use the word 'therapy' when the issues the client is endeavouring to tackle are particularly deepseated, reaching back into expectations and patterns created in childhood, whereas 'counselling' might be used to refer to work on more transient problems such as may arise from changes occurring in the client's life or crises in relationships. However, this distinction is not as neat as it looks, because a major part of the difficulty with changes or crises is that dealing with them will usually involve the client becoming aware of deep-seated expectations, patterns of relating and conflicts from earlier life which should properly be worked with by the practitioner whether she regards herself as a counsellor or therapist.
>
> (Mearns and Dryden 1990: x)

Third, centres identifying themselves as incorporating counselling and therapy from a feminist perspective are currently developing in Britain. This was the case at the Centre featured in this book.

Reflecting this degree of interchangeability, the term feminist therapy will therefore be used throughout as a shorthand term for the activity of feminist therapy and counselling. The women working at the Centre in question wished to be referred to as counsellors, therefore their wishes are respected. Employing the term counsellors, alongside feminist therapy as the generic term for their activities, hopefully represents the way in which both 'counselling' and 'therapy' inform feminist therapy.

Limitations to analysing women's emotional wellbeing solely in terms of subordination through gender

Gendered perspectives in contemporary feminist action

Work on elucidating the nature of women's emotional needs has both emanated from contemporary feminist action and helped to shape it. As specific issues relating to women's welfare have been addressed, so the case has been built up for defining the origins of what undermines women's emotional wellbeing as lying in social relations which construct, reproduce and reinforce women's subordination. The initial trigger for such a stand-point, or the corollary to it, is rejection of the pathologizing idea that women are intrinsically inferior. Thus, campaigning, support work in refuges and analysis concerned with domestic violence has shown that it is not a matter of isolated individual cases of the wayward wife or women addicted to violence 'bringing it on themselves'. Instead, such work has revealed that substantial populations of women across different class, age, health and ethnic backgrounds encounter physical violence and the concomitant psychological intimidation from male partners within the home. Attempts to enable women to escape individually and collectively from such coercion have revealed how powerfully entrenched in men's psyche, in organizations with a brief to protect personal welfare, and by default in the operation of the law and social policy, has been the belief that women are 'the appropriate victims of domestic violence' (Dobash and Dobash 1980, 1992; Binney, Harkell and Nixon 1981; Pahl 1985; Mama 1989).

As such accounts of the role of the social construction of gender in undermining women's emotional wellbeing have evolved, so a further feminist tradition has emerged. This is to treat 'emotional experience' as a permeable membrane, i.e. as being the site of interaction between various 'emotional' and 'non-emotional' factors. Women's feelings emerge as informed by the demands and possibilities arising from prevailing social conditions and the social and material resources these make available, by current ideological assumptions and by their attempts at self-expression engaging with these phenomena. Some of the gross inhumanity of pressures on women which constrain their self-expression in the first place are thus brought out. Furthermore, ways in which women's strategic attempts at self-expression in the face of such initial pressures are themselves subject to severe limitations and take possibly self-damaging forms are also explored. For example, in her work on women's coping strategies in poverty, Graham describes how in the face of the unremitting, under-resourced demands of childcare, women may turn to smoking as *the* available moment of emotional fulfilment in the day – and how even as they take their two to three minutes off they are still engaged in finding a way to do so which enables them to discharge the responsibilities of motherhood. 'Sometimes I put him outside the room, shut the door and put the radio on full blast and I've sat down and had a cigarette, calmed down and fetched him in again' (Graham 1993: 182).

Meanwhile, years of struggle and controversy – which still continues – has led to the understanding gaining ground that a variety of forms of oppression (as well as its gendered nature) are equally important in their effects on women's wellbeing. Black women have castigated white women feminists for their racism in assuming that gender is *the* common and central issue for women, irrespective of ethnic identity, and have organized around racism as an issue in its own right (Bryan and Dadzie 1985). Women experiencing physical disability have challenged able-bodied women to acknowledge that the subordinating effect of disablist attitudes is as powerful as that of sexist attitudes (Cross 1984; Morris 1991). Meanwhile, older women have brought the issue of ageist discrimination into play (Macdonald and Rich 1984).

As this understanding has grown, so has the appreciation that the state of any woman's emotional wellbeing may be shot through with the interplay of the effects of different social divisions. For example, Williams, on the multidimensional nature of the demands that mothers of young women with learning difficulties may face says

> in the study of black families' experiences in Lewisham, one mother of a child with special needs described feeling 'excluded' in her attempts to join in an all white parents self-help group. Ironically, such self-help groups are set up to protect parents, especially mothers, from the sense of isolation they already feel in having a disabled child. In this mother's case this sense of isolation was doubled.
>
> (Williams 1992: 161)

Feminist therapy – gender as the fulcrum of women's emotional wellbeing

Elements of analysis coalescing into the account of women's emotional wellbeing which has informed feminist therapy have developed along similar lines to that informing feminist action more generally. They have been characterized by attention to the social determinants of women's emotional wellbeing and its permeable nature. From an initial focus on the impact of gender, a more differentiated account has begun to develop.

The critique of the existing treatment of emotional disorders among women, which formed part of the initial impetus towards the development of feminist therapy, has been well rehearsed (see Gilbert 1980; Forisba 1981; Busfield 1989). Therefore it is summarized here. In keeping with feminist analyses of other spheres of women's experience, at its heart was an account of how women's emotional wellbeing was undermined by the sexism running throughout our social relations. It identified how, as a result of their social position, women's self-esteem was being eroded to the point of their experiencing profound and long-term states of anxiety and depression. As primary carers in the family, it was incumbent upon women constantly to devalue their own needs and interests. Meanwhile, although such work was regarded as essential, it was treated as being of secondary importance to men's role in public life. Moreover, any foray by women into public life was predestined to be viewed as inferior to what men could achieve. It was also seen either as a dereliction of familial duty, or as exceptional – and therefore likely to bring the woman to grief in some way (Forisba 1981).

Second, feminist commentators identified how women's emotional wellbeing was subject to a further blow as a result of the sexist nature of social relations. When women brought their 'complaints' to the mainly male medical and therapeutic practitioners, their morale was subverted by the treatment they received. They were responded to on the basis that the fault lay in their individual failure to adjust their circumstances and they were given palliatives such as tranquillizers to help them do so (Chesler 1972). Meanwhile, presentation for treatment confirmed the practitioners' existing frame of reference that women's mental health and capacity to cope was innately more feeble than men's (Broverman, Broverman, Clarkson et al. 1970). The scenario of 'male authority on emotional wellbeing, treating woman invalid', then provided an object lesson in male superiority as the solution and women's emotional frailty as the problem (Turkel 1976).

Developing out of this critique of the treatment of women in sexist society, writer/practitioners in feminist therapy have tried to map out to the furthest reaches of women's psyche how subordination through gender is at the fulcrum of women's emotional development. First, they have argued that assumptions and practices in society at large which treat women as subordinates filter into intrapsychic emotional processes that compose women's self-identity. Baker Miller writes:

> to concentrate on and to take seriously one's own development is hard enough for all human beings. But, as has been recently demonstrated in many areas, it has been even harder for women. In fact, women are encouraged to believe that if they do go through the mental and emotional struggle of self-development, the end result will be disastrous – they will forfeit the possibility of having any close relationships.
>
> (Baker Miller 1978: 20)

Such accounts have been complemented by analyses of women's emotional development as characterized by an intrapsychic experience of subordination *mediated by their interaction with significant others*. In numerous writings, Eichenbaum and Orbach, the co-founders of the first Women's Therapy

Centre in Britain, have set out how accounts of young women's emotional development centred on their relationship with their father, as in Freudian analysis, disregard the crucial relationship – that of the young woman with her mother. In doing so they have offered an analysis of the problematic nature for the young woman's emotional development of her relationship with her mother. They have posited that a young woman's emotional needs may be subordinated by her mother in various ways, ironically as an outcome of lifelong social pressures on the mother as a woman to treat her own emotional needs as secondary.

> As the mother transmits to her daughter the importance of caring for others, she brings to the relationship her *own* inner emotional needs. Inside each mother lives a hungry, needy, deprived and angry little girl. She turns to her daughter for nurturance, looking to the child to make up the loss of her own maternal nurturance.
>
> (Eichenbaum and Orbach 1985: 57)

Unconscious as well as conscious processes have been identified as active within this emotional universe. Again Eichenbaum and Orbach have identified unconscious processes as blocking women's self-expression. They have argued that as a result of coming up against the effect of unconscious processes in their work, they turned to Freudian analysis. This was because it offered the only existing description of such processes. 'The turn to psychoanalysis came from our new understanding of the importance of early family experience in forming our psychology' (1985: 13).

While doing so they have argued that they have been aware of tendencies within Freudian analysis to treat women's emotional development as centred on men's and secondary to it. Therefore they have described trying to retain the concept of the unconscious but with a feminist content: 'We saw the content of the unconscious as an intrapsychic reflection of the impact of present child-rearing and gender arrangements' (Eichenbaum and Orbach 1985: 14). They discuss how they have adopted interpretations within psychoanalytic work which they see as sensitive to women's emotional development as being important in its own right, and to interaction between women, i.e. mother and daughter, as playing a central role in this. Thus they have described using material from the work of Fairbairn (1952) Guntrip (1968) and Winnicott (1975) on the grounds that

> what they observed and what we shall be referring to is a model of psychological development in which what happens outside the womb and in earliest relationships is primary. We shall be talking mainly about the mother–child relationship because our culture has women mothering and for the most part being sole child rearers and care givers for infants and young children.
>
> (Eichenbaum and Orbach 1985: 14)

Decentring gender in feminist therapy

Gradually, in the theory informing feminist therapy, in parallel to feminist theorizing more generally, women's differential experience of social divisions other than gender, is being recognized as being as central to their emotional wellbeing. Existing work has been criticized for disregarding the diversity of women's experience. Brown, for example, has pinpointed how it has tended to reflect a 'Eurocentric bias'. In discussing Chernin's work on eating disorders (Chernin 1985) she comments as follows:

> an apt quote comes from Chernin. 'We are a unique generation of women – the first in history to have the social and psychological opportunity to surpass with ease the life choices our mothers have made' (p. 12). At this point one begins to nod in agreement – and yet must stop and ask, 'whose history? The history of which women, what mothers?' Such a statement may be true as regards a white middle-class, educationally privileged woman. How true is it for an American Indian woman living in a reservation community, the middle-class Black woman encountering barriers that while subtle are still obstacles to the full use of her education and professional development.
>
> (Brown 1990: 11)

Meanwhile, some therapists have focused on the impact of social divisions other than gender as central to understanding women's emotional wellbeing. For example, there are accounts from black women therapists in which they describe how they have focused on the impact of ethnicity and racism:

> for a black woman, seeing how we have internalised how society has decided what we are to be as Black women: we don't just look at the external as a political analysis would: we don't just look at the internal as a straight psychoanalytic, psychotherapist would, we look at the interaction between the two.
>
> (Laws 1991: 9)

Some therapists have also described trying to ensure that their understanding is informed by their own experience of oppression, by consciousness of the opportunities for solidarity that their own and other women's diverse experience may provide, while being sensitive to other women's experience of relative freedom from oppression which they may not share. Burstow on her practice:

> I have the knowledge that comes from being a Jew in an anti-semitic Christian centric world. I have the knowledge of being disabled and in physical pain in a world built for the able-bodied and the pain-free. And I have the knowledge that is forced on you when you are a woman with a woman's partner in this lesbophobic society . . . I am also white. I know

that having white privilege distorts my vision ... As a counsellor teacher, supervisor and writer I have been struggling to access other vision ... From the opposite side, I know as well that the very oppressions to which I am subject sometimes blind me to the experiences of women on the opposite side of that oppression.

(Burstow 1992: xvii)

Despite the development of the standpoint within feminist therapy that women's differential experience of social divisions is central to their emotional wellbeing, such awareness is still far from suffusing its current analysis. For example, Walker's account published in 1990 and drawing on her own experience as a practitioner can still argue in the following generic terms:

to understand the position and experiences of women today it is necessary to know something of their history. Women do not exist in a vacuum, they are influenced by a society that both implicitly and explicitly gives messages about their expected and accepted role and position.

(Walker 1990: 22)

Meanwhile, the dearth of accounts from women participating in feminist therapy also limits evidence of the importance of this issue in their experience. Therefore it is crucial to explore how the impact of a range of social inequalities informs the experience of women coming to feminist therapy.

Exploring the limitations to analysing women's emotional wellbeing in terms of subordination through gender

Primary personal relationships

This book treats accounts of primary personal relationships as sensitive indicators of the impact of social divisions on women's emotional wellbeing. In feminist practice and writing, what are conventionally defined as primary personal relationships – such as those with parents and male partners – have emerged paradoxically and tragically as one site where women's emotional welfare is undermined in a gendered way. For example, feminist analysis has unveiled the endemic nature of father–daughter sexual abuse and its harrowing emotional consequences for the young women concerned (Ward 1984). In addition to work on domestic violence (Yllö and Bograd 1988), feminist research has chronicled the myriad ways in which relationships with male partners have tended to erode women's emotional wellbeing. For example, Hemmings, writing on older women's accounts of marriage:

> some of the contributors chronicle a sharing of love, care, responsibilities: most tell of agonizing incompatibilities, or a give and take which turned out mainly at the women's expense. Even in reasonably 'good' marriages, women describe how they have for years suppressed their own needs and intellect in order to preserve their husband's sense of self.
>
> (Hemmings 1985: 7)

Meanwhile, for example in in-depth studies of women's experience of parenting in relative poverty, feminist analysis has begun to give an account of the way in which other dimensions to social inequality may suffuse women's experience of such relationships to the detriment of women's emotional wellbeing. Here, as in Conway's account of homeless women, parenting in bed and breakfast accommodation, the near impossibility in such conditions of women meeting what are defined as parental responsibilities, let alone providing for their own emotional wellbeing, is what is so destructive in its effects:

> Sheila and her 14-month-old daughter live in a room approximately 7 feet by 15 feet. The small window is at least six feet high up on the wall and gives very little light. As there is no room for a cot, the daughter shares Sheila's bed and disturbs her through the night. The hotel has no kitchen and food is not allowed in the rooms. Sheila does not even have a kettle to make a hot drink. She is often hungry, but worries more about her daughter who is often ill and does not seem to be growing.
>
> (Conway 1988: 41)

The emotional stress experienced by women in this situation was revealed in their comments. Out of the 56 women interviewed, 44 said they were unhappy most of the time, 41 were tired most of the time, 35 often lost their temper, 34 often couldn't sleep at night, 33 said their children got on top of them and 24 said they burst into tears for no reason (Conway 1988: 44).

Therefore, accounts from women participating in feminist therapy of what they identified as primary personal relationships and their positive and negative impact on their emotional wellbeing, seem likely to reflect the range of social inequalities in play.

The selective nature of our sample

As our sample came from women drawn to a feminist therapy centre (hereafter the Centre), it was characterized by the circumstances of the population of women the Centre attracted. There was therefore the danger that paradoxically, discrimination or disadvantage at work in restricting access to the Centre might yield muted evidence of its effects in interaction with gender in women's accounts. Women who experienced these effects might either not appear in our sample or in very small numbers (Brown 1990). In fact this was borne out by the way in which our sample (see Appendix 2) reflected the general pattern of very few older women or non-White women engaging in practice at the Centre (see Appendix 1).

The significance of children's comparative powerlessness

The way in which children's emotional needs may be subordinated and denied in our existing social relations as a reflection of their comparative powerlessness is an important dimension to inequality in its own right (Miller 1988, 1989; Valentine 1989; Ryan and Stubbs 1989). Because of this and to counteract the risk that the impact of social inequalities, other than gender, might be played down because of the selective nature of the population coming to the Centre, we paid close attention to the possible impact of women's comparative powerlessness as children on their emotional well-being in childhood and subsequently. We had accounts of childhood experience from *all* the women. Moreover, such experience was likely to have been recalled and therefore readily retrievable as a result of women's contact with the Centre. Even if such experience had not been considered in terms of children's structural powerlessness as a group, it was likely to have been examined. Theories informing feminist psychotherapy have focused on the influential nature of childhood interactions – albeit as *characterized by the operation of gender* – in shaping young women's emotional development at the time and subsequently (Eichenbaum and Orbach 1984).

The possibility of disaggregating the effects of children's comparative powerlessness and gender, and the importance of doing so to clarify the effects of both, is illustrated in the following extract from Spring's autobiographical account. Her father's physical abuse of her may have been gendered in nature. However, it is clearly adult parental authority which reinforces the silence between the two children, destroying any chance of solidarity.

> I can remember sitting with my brother David in the garden, wanting to tell him that my father was touching me in a way I hated . . . In the end I couldn't do it. Extraordinary as it may seem, we were both so imbued with family propaganda that it seemed traitorous to even think, much less talk rebelliously. Neither of us could mention misery. We were not supposed to be miserable.
>
> (Spring 1987: 53)

Given that the women's accounts were retrospective following feminist therapy, there is a danger that women may have been encouraged to over-emphasize the importance of childhood experience, albeit as proof of the influence of the gendered nature of social relations. In this way their accounts may have been distorted. In the event, there were two safeguards against this. First, women's accounts clarified whether the impact of childhood events led them to feminist therapy. Second, women were aware of and referred to the counsellors' emphasis and bias.

Treatment of social divisions

The degrees of inequality and difference discussed here, seemingly so intrinsic to society that they constitute part of its structures, are not treated simplistically in the course of analysis as determining events. Instead, an attempt is made to discern the degree to which they are implicated in events and responses to them – and consequently how influential in the constitution of women's emotional wellbeing they may be considered to be.

Post-structuralist and post-modernist theories have also reached feminist social work – my own field (see Langan 1992). They stress the infinite diversity and changeability of experience, how in turn its nature is relative to constantly changing perceptions of it and how in turn these perceptions are relative to each other (Weedon 1987). In contrast, referring to fundamental divisions in society as characterizing experience, as I have done, can seem rather ponderous. However, the suffering that results from such inequalities means that it is important not to retreat from trying to give some account of their effects. Nevertheless, while analysing women's accounts, the fluid nature of the power relations women were living through and of their own perceptions became apparent. Therefore an attempt is made to reflect this fluidity.

Beyond subordination alone

Besides considering the limitations of accounts of women's wellbeing couched solely in terms of its gendered nature, this book also considers the limitations to analysing women's emotional wellbeing in terms of its *subordinated* nature alone.

Lawrence's work indicates that practitioners of feminist therapy do encounter and recognize the existence of women's capacity for self-expression – albeit hideously distorted and undermined. This is reflected in her account of a young woman whose anorexia in an otherwise well-running life seemed a mystery.

it was when I asked her what it was she liked about working with small children that she began to become confused. It was not a question of *what* she liked about the work. She had never even thought about whether she liked it at all. Why did she choose to be friends with some girls rather than others? Again, the puzzled look. Alison did not choose friends; she waited to be chosen. What did she especially enjoy about geography and history? In truth, she never really thought about that either. She had been told she was good at them so she *did* them.

Here was a young women whose life was really out of control. Everything was well planned, but by whom? The only aspect of life which she could really control was her size and shape.

(Lawrence 1984: 101)

Despite such awareness, analysis informing feminist therapy has tended to treat the extinction of women's capacity for self-expression, through its subordination, as the fulcrum of women's emotional identity. This is reflected in the following account from Eichenbaum and Orbach:

Mother and all those who relate to the girl, respond to and develop in her all those capacities that will fit her psychologically for her future social role . . . Attachment to and concern for others becomes her guide . . . She begins to identify the satisfying of others' needs, and complying with others, as a need of her own . . .

(Eichenbaum and Orbach 1988: 52)

However, there is no corresponding analysis which would account for why women become unhappy as a result and do not simply enter a state of emotional quietude and acceptance if their capacity for self-expression is so subordinated. Nor is women's espousal of a feminist analysis and approach or the determination to gain relief through feminist therapy accounted for. As Ryan has commented:

We now have an extensive understanding of how we unconsciously reproduce our mothers' oppression . . . what we also need to do is understand how we do not only do this: how we have managed to rebel, to be different, to become feminists.

(Ryan 1983)

This book aims to take account of how women's capacity for self-expression and assertiveness characterizes their emotional wellbeing, as well as the tendency for this to be subordinated. Otherwise there is a danger of distorting the nature of women's emotional resources, what has happened to them, and their potential.

A further dimension to the nature of women's emotional wellbeing, which is neglected by analysis rooted solely in the idea of gender subordination, is women's capacity for dominating behaviour. The absence of discussion of this can still characterize texts concerned with feminist therapy, e.g. Walker (1990). However, appreciation of the fact that women's behaviour can be

mediated by social divisions other than gender has opened up acknowledgement in feminist debate that women can behave in a dominating way.
For example, the way in which women not experiencing learning difficulties
have disregarded the needs and interests of women who do has been put on
record (see Williams 1992). This book therefore tries to take account of this
dimension to women's behaviour from their accounts.

How egalitarian are the theories counsellors work to and the activities instituted in feminist therapy?

The impetus of self-help

The critique of the sexist nature of women's emotional wellbeing and of sexist
responses to it was important in the original development of feminist therapy.
However, it did not alone provide the creative spark behind its emergence.
There could have been a legion of such critiques without one network of
feminist therapists or feminist therapy centres arising. The crucial step was
provided by the self-help approach: women deciding that they did not accept
that what exists by way of treatment of women's emotional problems is all
that can be. Instead they have created their own resources aimed at meeting
women's emotional needs on their own terms. In this respect the development
of feminist therapy parallels developments in contemporary feminist action
more generally. Feminist self-help initiatives have provided a forum in which
women have felt free to explore the emotional injuries arising from the
operation of gender, because by definition such problems are not ascribed to
their personal inadequacy. This process is illustrated by the experience of
participants in such a group discussing women's health problems:

> We're talking about health problems that particularly affect women,
> which range not only from menstrual difficulties and childbirth and
> postnatal depression, but just general depression and anxiety, which
> more and more of us are realising now is a result of the situation we're in
> . . . and that it's not a particular weakness in women.
>
> (Donnelly 1986)

The experience of such initiatives, whatever their scale, is that change on
the part of social institutions in relation to the issues they are addressing is at
best very slow (Curno, Lamming, Leach et al. 1982). Nevertheless, women's
accounts of their involvement in feminist self-help initiatives indicate that the
way women's emotional needs are subordinated is not an immutable social
construction. Such initiatives are on record as the locations where, however
fleetingly, women demonstrate their capacity to begin to create social
conditions that meet rather than subvert their emotional needs. To refer back
to the women's health group, one of the participants went on to comment:

'it's magic really that it's the women's groups that are actually breaking through that sort of blanket of depression on the estate . . .' (Donnelly 1986).

How the development of feminist therapy reflects this self-help drive, comes across in the account of the establishment of the Women's Therapy Centre in Britain, by its two founders:

> On the morning of April 6, 1976, we deposited a hundred envelopes in the mailbox outside Chalk Farm Tube Station, London. In each was a letter and a leaflet announcing the opening of The Women's Therapy Centre in Islington on April 8. The mailing went to women's groups, women's centres, doctors in the area, educational institutions, psychiatric clinics and national and local media . . . Friends came to help and we chatted excitedly about our plans for the Centre. We were opening it, we said, because women wanted psychotherapeutic services that addressed women's needs, understood women's experience and supported women's struggles.
>
> (Eichenbaum and Orbach 1985: Preface)

These developments do not owe their existence only to the initiative of women who have wanted to practise therapy from a feminist perspective. They could not have come into being without women who wanted help with emotional problems, either choosing to work in self-help groups with other women or starting to reject male therapists, as the personification of sexist attitudes to women. The growth of the wider women's movement was crucial in bringing this process about. For example, Turkel, a women therapist writing in 1976 in the United States, noted a change in women's attitude to the therapist's sex. She described how previously women would tend to choose a male therapist in preference to a female because they were following the social norm of assuming men had superior competence as professionals. More recently in her experience, women had been demanding women therapists in preference to men because they saw women therapists as sharing understanding of the social disadvantages women faced: 'They perceive men as hostile to women and as not wanting women to achieve' (Turkel 1976: 120).

Emphasis on equality within feminist therapy

The corollary to the self-help ethos which marked the emergence of feminist therapy was the emphasis on an egalitarian approach to relations between women as therapists and participants. Women therapists and participants were identified as sharing a common knowledge base in relation to women's emotional wellbeing, derived from their experience of the sexist nature of social relations (Sturdivant 1980). Considerable attention was also devoted to trying to create a relationship of equality between therapist and participant. The main strategies employed to achieve this have been identified by Watson and Williams in their reviews of early practice, as feminist therapists: attempting to clarify the process of their work to participants; making their personal standpoint explicit; prompting participants' rights, e.g. over choice of a therapist in a Centre; encouraging participants to negotiate the aims and evaluate the outcome of therapy; and emphasizing participants' strengths (Watson and Williams 1992: 218).

Diversity of approach to practice

While reflecting this egalitarian intent, the development of feminist therapy has not been characterized by the growth of uniform practice. Organizationally, in the USA and Britain, feminist therapy has not been controlled by bureaucratic regulating bodies. It has been composed of an interactive network composed of individuals concerned with developing and/or benefiting from the practice and ideas involved, communicating through meetings, conferences, publications, registers and centres (Brown and Liss-Levinson 1981; Ernst and Maguire 1987; Heenan 1988).

Women have also developed the practice of feminist therapy while coming from differing backgrounds in counselling or therapy. So, for example, at a conference for women in the field of feminist therapy organized by British Women's Therapy Centres I attended, the platform was shared by women who identified themselves respectively as humanistic, psychoanalytic, eclectic and art therapists, though all were seeking to work out how such practice and a feminist perspective might mesh together.

Despite such diversity, women practising in feminist therapy can be discerned as drawing, in the main, on two areas of practice (see Ernst and Maguire 1987; Walker 1990; Burstow 1992). These are a psychotherapeutic approach and the approach embodied in humanistic/person centred counselling. Even so, there are clearly different tendencies in the way in which these two schools of practice conceptualize the development of women's emotional state and problems arising in relation to it. Feminist therapy informed by a psychotherapeutic approach locates primary influences on emotional development as lying in the nature of maternal–infant relations in infancy, with formative effects on the impact of women's unconscious state, which, in turn, inhibit conscious thought and actions. The route to revising this process lies through these unconscious inhibitions being raised to consciousness and being rendered amenable to challenge. This is seen as being brought about by the support of an other (or others), aware of the existence of such processes, and encouraging the individual women concerned by refraining from rejecting her whatever the nature of the perceptions that emerge from her unconscious.

By contrast, in feminist therapy informed by humanistic or 'person-centred' counselling (Rogers 1961), the focus is on how the individual woman has currently within herself all the resources for meeting her own emotional needs, but that their expression is inhibited by the hostile nature of current interpersonal and social relations. The route to the woman concerned realizing these emotional resources and enjoying their benefits is by her being provided with a relationship in counselling characterized by for instance 'unconditional positive regard', which does not obstruct her fulfilling her emotional potential.

Feminist therapy has also been characterized by a variety of modes of practice ranging from one-to-one work between an identified therapist/ counsellor and client, to either groups led by therapists or counsellors, or self-help groups, to co-counselling where the roles of counsellor and counselled are shared in turn (see Ernst and Goodison 1981; Ernst and Maguire 1987).

Meanwhile some therapists and centres have also tried to organize their practice around the recognition that other social divisions than gender are as central to women's emotional wellbeing: for example, the Shanti Therapy Centre in Britain, funded through the National Health Service. Shanti has provided free, brief psychotherapy to women with its local catchment area.

> The workers are all women, but diverse in other respects – in culture, ethnicity, age and sexuality. Shanti prioritises women who would have difficulty getting good access to other services; ethnic minority women, lesbians, older women, working-class women and women with disabilities.
>
> (Laws 1991: 9)

A common focus of practice

Despite all these different tendencies, practice informing feminist therapy shares two characteristics which also mark it out from other feminist initiatives. First, although women's emotional state is regarded as permeable, i.e. susceptible to the influence of social conditions more generally, emphasis is laid on its also being an entity in its own right. Ryan discusses the way in which any therapeutic approach reflects the fact that people inhabit a social and material world and 'an internal world of their own mental and psychic structure'. She then argues that feminist therapy has a 'concern to understand internal and external reality together ... in a way that recognizes how external reality forms and oppresses women, at the same time as understanding the autonimity and powerfulness of internal reality' (Ryan 1983: 11).

Conceptualizing women's emotional state as an entity in its own right can be seen as legitimating the second distinctive characteristic of the practice of feminist therapy. This is to treat this entity – this internal state – as *the* site for intervention, in order to promote women's emotional wellbeing. These two characteristics are displayed in Ernst and Goodison's account of the development of their practice rooted in psychotherapy.

> Unconscious feelings formed by our childhood conditioning would continue to sabotage our conscious choices for liberation. Recognising that we needed to unlearn this conditioning, we started to bring to the surface some of our repressed feelings. This process should perhaps have been called 'unconsciousness raising' . . . We hoped that by making the unconscious conscious we would reveal the ways in which we had absorbed and internalised the prevailing ideology. We could then, uncover, root out and deal with those recalcitrant feelings to gain control of our emotional lives and direct them more effectively.
>
> (Ernst and Goodison 1981: 4)

They then contrast this practice with what they define as feminist practice in other spheres.

> Our experience showed us that real change would come from *combining* our political activity in the world with the ideas and experience coming from discussion and consciousness raising groups *and* with the feelings and emotional energy we can tap through therapy.
>
> (Ernst and Goodison 1981: 4)

Walker's account of feminist practice derived from humanistic or person-centred counselling reflects the same two characteristics – 'Encouraging women to trust themselves, to become more assertive and to be able to acknowledge and express anger are other central themes in feminist work' (Walker 1990: 75).

This approach is also discernible in feminist therapy informed by more of a minority interest in practice – art therapy.

> Natural mediums, such as water, mud, clay and sand, provide space for self exploration, can trigger connections between influences in present relationships and past patterns, or provide echoes of past and current attitudes to body image.
>
> (Butler and Wintram 1991: 55)

Critique of the egalitarian nature of feminist therapy's approach

Despite the egalitarian intent of feminist therapy's analysis and practice, there has been a battery of criticism suggesting that it has inherent shortcomings, which mean it is unlikely to resolve the inequalities implicated in women's emotional distress. First, there has been concern that there is a disjuncture between the feminist analysis informing feminist therapy and the nature of its therapeutic and counselling practice. For example, Dobash and Dobash argue that in feminist therapy, despite the origins of women's emotional suffering being identified as stemming from prevailing social conditions, in practice this is treated as lying in a masochistic tendency on the part of individual women to subordinate their own interests. False hope of a solution to the problem of emotional suffering is then given by encouraging women to reverse this trend in counselling and therapy, so that they will be able to 'take on the world' more positively, thereby reducing the likelihood of further suffering on their own part. This whole process is also seen as having the pathologizing effect of defining emotional suffering as rooted in problems in the individual women's personality (Dobash and Dobash 1992: Ch. 7).

Second, despite the self-help ethos of feminist therapy, the counsellor–client relationship has been viewed as intrinsically hierarchical. For example, Ussher asserts:

> The notion of an equal relationship in feminist therapy is also problematic, for how egalitarian and equal can any therapy be? One person is paid, is secure, has knowledge and training. The other is distressed, often frightened and needing help. This can never be an equal relationship, and to pretend that it is may actually be disempowering as it pays lipservice to egalitarian practice, without fundamentally changing anything.
>
> (Ussher 1991: 235)

If this is the case, it can be seen as giving rise to the danger that women in feminist therapy may defer to the counsellors' view of the nature of their problems, as opposed to being able at last to express what these are, in an uninhibited way, thereby gaining some true resolution of them.

Third, the degree to which the forms of organization created in feminist therapy are models of equity, i.e. meeting – not subordinating – women's needs, has also been raised.

> There is nothing inherently 'feminist' about any one organisational structure . . . For example, the goal of collective self-management may be a 'feminist' one in the context of a consciousness raising group, or a self-help group, since it is the structure that can most effectively express the (feminist) aspirations of the women concerned. It is not, however, necessarily 'feminist' when adopted by a voluntary organisation set up to meet women's needs, since it offers no means for those women concerned as users to express their demands (through a management committee, for example).
>
> (Sturdy 1987: 39–40)

Moreover, as raised earlier, criticism has also been directed, not so much against the modes of practice and organization of feminist therapy, as against the fact that it tends not to take account of the range of sources of oppression in women's life, other than the gendered nature of social relations.

Exploring the egalitarian nature of the theories counsellors work to and the activities instituted in feminist therapy

The counsellors' standpoint

This book presents empirical evidence on the validity of the existing critique of feminist therapy. The accounts from the group of counsellors at the Centre are reviewed, to reveal the extent to which their analysis of the constituent elements in women's emotional wellbeing reflects understanding of the impact of a range of profound social inequalities, as exemplified in women's accounts of their own lives. Then – although the fuller answer to this obviously draws on women's accounts – the book explores the degree to which the counsellors' accounts yield evidence of how non-hierarchical are the power relations between them and women participants in the organiz- ation and practice of feminist therapy. The impact of the organization and practice of the Centre on the counsellors' and coordinators' own wellbeing is also considered, including whether it reproduces the scenario of the demands of women's care of others, undermining their own welfare (Graham 1984). Finally, it is important to put counsellor's intentions in relation to theory and practice on the record in their own right. These may emerge as entirely defensible, but undermined in the event by inclement conditions, such as the necessity for stringent rationing of scarce available resources (Sturdy 1987).

The representative nature of work at the Centre

As commented on earlier, feminist therapy has developed in an eclectic way, characterized by diversity in theory and approaches to practice. Therefore, the practice of a specific network or centre cannot crudely be taken as representative of its totality. Nevertheless, although the counsellors were a small group (four), their work at the Centre reflected a background in both psychotherapy and counselling. It also incorporated a further variety of influences – such as Gestalt therapy (see Perls 1976, and Note 1, end of Chapter 4); and Transactional Analysis (see Berne 1961, 1968). Similarly to other centres of feminist therapy, different modes of practice were under- taken at the Centre: one-to-one counselling, group work, specific workshops. Moreover, the counsellors had indicated a commitment to addressing women's experience of different social divisions. As the Centre in question was not the original site of feminist therapy in Britain it also provided the opportunity to sample the nature of practice as it spread across the country. In its own right it was also a focus for practice across a wide area. In these ways practice at the Centre can be seen as reflecting to some degree both the variety of work embodied in feminist therapy more generally and some of its main tendencies, and therefore provides the opportunity to consider the issues arising from these.

Moreover, the way in which the counsellors and coordinator in question participated in our study opened up the possibility of probing the nature of practice in some depth. The counsellors agreed to our interviewing women participants who had been the subject of the work on which the counsellors had been interviewed. Therefore the experience of counsellors and clients concerning the same practice can be put together. The counsellors were also prepared to discuss the relationship of their professional practice to their personal life. This means that some idea of its impact on their own emotional wellbeing can be gained. We were also able to interview the whole team of workers including the administrative coordinator, whose work embodies responsibility for administrative, secretarial and reception duties but not specifically therapeutic practice. It was seen in the Centre as of equal importance to the work of the counsellors and thereby provides an important test of how well non-hierarchical organizational principles work in practice.

In common with other centres of feminist therapy, the work did not all hinge on the efforts of individual counsellors. There were workshops run by other practitioners under its aegis. While sampling counselling together with group work, we nevertheless concentrated on examining the practice and experience of the counsellors. Their efforts were primarily responsible for initiating policy and gaining and maintaining resources. Therefore examining these is crucial to understanding the theories and practices that inform the development of feminist therapy in this location.

How egalitarian are the outcomes of feminist therapy?

Issues for consideration

The existing critique of feminist therapy raises a number of disturbing questions concerning the degree to which the egalitarian intent of feminist therapy is realized in practice. This critique clearly has implications for assessing the outcomes of feminist therapy. However, there are two further issues which the development of feminist therapy raises, which it is crucial to address in assessing the degree to which its outcomes amount to a more equitable experience of emotional wellbeing. First, even if feminist therapy is able to produce some relief from emotional distress, how thorough-going is this relief if intervention is confined to an individual woman's emotional state, but widespread social conditions implicated in women's emotional suffering are left unresolved?

One case in point is the relationship of feminist therapy to conditions of relative poverty. In addition to the undermining effects on women's emotional wellbeing of parenting in poverty, discussed earlier, relative poverty is heavily implicated in women's emotional suffering generally. For example, epidemiological studies such as Blaxter's using self-defined concepts of psychological wellbeing have found a significant relationship between low incomes among women of all ages and 'the likelihood of greater malaise' (Blaxter 1990: 71–2). The rate at which women consult GPs for mental health problems also reveals that women from lower occupational groups, are over one-third more likely to consult than women in classes I and II (OPCS 1990).

Without otherwise altering such conditions, the support provided through access to a confiding relationship has been identified in its own right as having some protective effect (Blaxter 1990: 229), and in warding off the onset of depression (Wing and Bebbington 1982). Feminist therapy might be able to provide just such a relationship and therefore some relief from emotional suffering. Initiatives like the Shanti Centre (Laws 1991) and more generally the work that Holland has helped to pioneer (Holland 1989, 1990, 1992) have also deliberately set out to reach women living in relative poverty and to tackle the affects of poverty on their emotional wellbeing through counselling and therapy. Accounts of this practice argue that women gain some relief as a result. They also provide evidence that some women have gained a sufficient sense of solidarity and feel robust enough to organize a similar service for other women locally on a self-help basis (Holland 1989, 1990, 1992).

However, even such activism leaves the widespread nature of women's relative poverty untouched. Complex and wide ranging social changes seem necessary to relieve it. These include measures relating to income redistribution generally (Quick and Wilkinson 1991) and measures to alter conditions which depress women's chances in the labour market, such as unequal educational opportunities and expectations of women's responsibilities as informal carers (Payne 1991). Feminist therapy does not embody such measures. Therefore, how full can the relief provided by counselling and therapy be said to be for the individual women experiencing relative poverty, while such conditions grind on untouched?

Unless the question of the degree of relief which feminist therapy can bring (without touching widespread social conditions implicated in undermining women's emotional well-being) is broached, the scale of its achievement is obscure, and the extent to which women should invest their energies in it is unclear.

A further major issue omitted from analysis of the outcomes of feminist therapy is the extent to which it results in reinforcing women's capacity for dominating behaviour. The tendency not to conceptualize women's behaviour in such terms, as discussed earlier, may mean that such an issue does not get explicit attention in its practice. However, it is clearly important in considering the egalitarian nature of its outcomes.

Making headway on the question of the outcomes of feminist therapy is also impossible without evidence from women participants on the following matters: To what extent do women experience the undermining effects of current social relations on their emotional welfare as being resolved in the course of feminist therapy and as a result of it? Are the outcomes of feminist therapy oppressive to others' interests in any way? Such evidence is offered here through women's accounts of their experience of feminist therapy.

Exploring the egalitarian nature of the outcomes of feminist therapy

Why women come to feminist therapy is explored first to unravel the nature of the emotional problems and resources women bring to it, its attractions, and the extent to which these reflect the impact of social inequalities. From the women's accounts, what they see as having a positive effect on their emotional wellbeing is then established, together with the nature of this effect and how they see it coming about. Any negative aspects of their experience of the organization of the Centre and interaction while there are also discussed. In the course of doing so, the women's views of all these processes are compared with those of the counsellors. Where the outcome of engaging in feminist therapy is positive as far as the women in question are concerned, this experience is still critiqued. Without denying the reality of women's experience, it can nevertheless emerge as having negative consequences or limitations.

Interviewing arrangements

Women currently engaged in therapy were not interviewed. On ethical grounds interviewing in the course of feminist therapy might unwittingly have intruded in a way which would have had a negative effect on the interactions in progress (Gilbert 1980). Pragmatically it might also have been extremely difficult to deduce whether unresolved issues were due to the stage or the quality of the work. Women were interviewed at least six months after they had ceased contact with the Centre. First, this offered some chance of discerning how the results of feminist therapy fared as they became interwoven with other events in women's lives while women were without continuing contact with the Centre. Second, it meant that women's recall of why they had gone to the Centre and what contact had been like might still be vivid.

Nature of women's contact with the Centre

The experience of women in the sample represents work on the part of all the counsellors at the Centre. It also reflects the range of lengths of time women were in contact with the Centre, in order to convey a sense of the issues that the timescale of contact in counselling and therapy raises. It is not necessarily the case that women facing the most deepseated problems have the longest time in feminist therapy. However, contact ranged from one interview to three years (see Appendix 2) and to some degree this was seen by the women themselves and the counsellors as reflecting the nature of the problems they faced. Women had a variety of forms of involvement with the Centre. The aim is to reflect this variety – although in some instances the numbers are small – and draw on experience of one-to-one counselling of varying lengths, of one-off assessment interviews which were the most numerous form of contact and group work.

Working with women at the Centre

Within the limits of our resources, and because we were concerned to do justice to the depth and nuances of women's experience in their relationships generally (and more specifically in feminist therapy), we concentrated on gaining fuller accounts from a smaller number of women, rather than more superficial accounts or written returns from larger numbers.

While retaining our independent view of the Centre and its work, it was important that both of us carrying out interviewing gained some understanding of the demands and possibilities of engaging first hand in feminist therapy which were authentic in relation to our own situation at the time. Therefore we both had initial assessment interviews (see Chapter 4 for a fuller account of their place in the work of the Centre) and we used them to explore emotional demands and dilemmas we were facing. I also participated in some groupwork as part of the Centre's workshop programme.

In contributing to the work on which this book is based, women participants discussed experiences which had been sources of happiness for them, but often experiences which had also had searing effects. Doing so required considerable bravery. It was also courageous of the counsellors and coordinator to open up their practice to such public inspection. Both groups participated on the basis that this might help other women. Hopefully this book does justice to their efforts.

two	

Kept in the family: women's emotional wellbeing in childhood relationships

Introduction

A major theme in literature relating to feminist therapy is the primary role of gender in undermining women's emotional welfare. The mother–daughter relationship in childhood has also been seen as central to this process, notably in the work of Eichenbaum and Orbach.

They have argued that women introject the idea that it is right that they put their emotional needs second to those of others.

> The first psychological demand that follows from a woman's social role is that she must defer to others, follow their lead, articulate her needs only in relation to theirs . . . As a result of this social requirement women come to believe that they are not important in themselves. Women come to feel that they are unworthy, undeserving and unenriched.
>
> (Eichenbaum and Orbach 1982: 29)

They have also identified the mother–daughter relationship as the crucial vehicle for bringing this about: 'She [her mother] teaches her to look after others. The daughter, as she learns to hide her needy little-girl part, becomes extremely sensitive to neediness in others . . . *she learns to give what others need*' (Eichenbaum and Orbach 1985: 56). This involves the woman as daughter, learning to put her mother's (otherwise unmet) emotional needs before her own. 'As the daughter learns her role as nurturer *her first child is her mother*' (Eichenbaum and Orbach 1985: 57).

Our findings modify and move beyond this thesis in several ways. They indicate that for the women in our sample, in childhood the gendered nature of their existence had undermined their emotional wellbeing. However, the women had not accepted their mother's treatment of them, but had been critical of it – demonstrating a capacity for assertiveness and self-expression. The nature of their relationship with their fathers had also been important in its own right. Moreover, the interplay of a number of dimensions to social inequality, including their comparative lack of power as children, had been reflected in their emotional wellbeing. In connection with their comparative lack of power as children, the fact that their capacity to give as well as receive affection had lacked recognition, had been an important factor.

Participation in feminist therapy was the one known common point of the experience of the women concerned. Otherwise their personal circumstances were diverse. Their ages ranged from mid-fifties to early twenties, so their childhoods occurred across a broad time-scale ending about ten years previously. This meant that features that could have come across strongly from the experience of cohorts of children of similar ages or from systematically selected backgrounds might not have done so in this group. Nevertheless, certain consistent themes emerged from women's perceptions of their childhood. At the same time, the ways in which these themes were tempered pointed to further important dimensions of childhood experience.

In terms of ethnic identity, one woman's (Gillian's) ethnic identity was British born African-Caribbean and that of her parents and stepfather African-Caribbean. The ethnic identity of Nina and her family was White continental European. Otherwise the ethnic identity of the group and their parents was White British. Women identified themselves as coming from comfortably off or relatively poor backgrounds in childhood. Their comments concentrate on childhood experience as opposed to adolescence, as they were invited to focus on their earlier years, to clarify influential factors in their experience then.

The retrospective nature of this study meant we could not know whether or not the women's accounts were different from what they would have said before feminist therapy. However, it was possible to pick up and take account of some of the ways in which its influence was discernible or noticeable by its absence. Its influence on women's perspectives also raised significant issues in its own right for their emotional wellbeing.

Relationships with mothers and women's capacity for assertiveness and self-expression

In describing how through their mother's influence, young women come to put the needs of others first, Eichenbaum and Orbach depict young women as being enveloped in their mother's psychological universe, not only as an integral part of their identity – but prior to a distinct self-identity forming.

Before the baby 'knows' itself as a person, with a distinct inside and outside, before it can distinguish itself from the people and objects around it, it exists in a merged state with mother. Just as, prior to birth it lived within the actual boundaries of mother's body so after birth it lives within the mother's psychological boundaries. The mother sets up a psychological milieu that the two inhabit. To put it more precisely, the aspects of the mother, that are preoccupied with caring for the infant, and the infant in its entirety, live within this psychological framework.

(Eichenbaum and Orbach 1988: 48)

Later, still speaking of the young woman:

she has learnt directly and indirectly, in this first important relationship with her mother, that attachment to others – a prerequisite of survival – depends upon two features.
1. The repression of her own 'needing to be developed' selfhood and
2. an almost compulsive concern for others. Thus attachment as she knows it, is itself problematic. For it is characterised by repression and merger. It goes hand in hand with the loss of a personal identity.

(Eichenbaum and Orbach 1988: 53)

What seems to be described here is the all-pervasive influence of one human being on the self-identity of the other. Our findings are not consistent with this picture.

Women in our sample had not simply introjected the idea through interaction with their mothers, that it was right that their emotional needs were not met, thereby emerging with the 'women's psychology' Eichenbaum and Orbach have postulated. This is demonstrated in several ways: first by the way in which women had been *critical* of their mother's treatment of them and of the way in which their mothers had not met their emotional needs. *Gillian*: 'I had no love – my mum loved me but not the way I wanted. I wanted her to show she loved me.' *Debbie* of her mother: 'No physical love. That may come down to the fact she had four kids in close succession, and she had a difficult childhood, which made it hard for her to show affection.' Women consistently identified their mothers as having provided the main source of day-to-day care of their physical needs. However many of the women had not felt that their mother's efforts in this respect had been successful in meeting their emotional needs.

Nina: The way she showed she loved us was through actually making sure we were well fed, that we were dressed in clean clothes, all the physical things of looking after. But I don't remember ever having a hug from her. I don't even know if I did but I can't remember it.

Zoë commented on her mother as follows: 'Mother obviously loved us but she wasn't overtly loving. She was always very cross.'

Even where the women described their mothers as having come closer to meeting their emotional needs, their responses indicated this was an issue they had weighed up in childhood, instead of simply acquiescing in how they were treated. *Mary* contrasted her aunt, whom she also identified as one of the most important people to her in childhood, with her mother. Her aunt had brought up three sons alone, was very independent and had to work. Her mother, on the other hand, was

> completely the opposite . . . very caring . . . in to the role of feeding us and looking after us . . . we had such a lot of respect for her . . . because my father ruled. She had to be there. 'Get the meals . . . or there'd be a row.' She wasn't allowed to work. I didn't understand that then.

Christine described her mother as caring but very soft, also passive. Her mother had had many arguments with Christine's grandmother in which she had always had to back down. 'Softness equated weakness for me', said Christine. *Esther*, on her mother: 'She just gave me what I wanted, basically. I remember it being warm and nice, we weren't well off . . . I remember it as being a really happy childhood.'

Women's accounts also reflected how taking on gendered caretaking roles as young women could be marked by reluctance on their part and not simply by acceptance.

> *Katherine*: With my dad I always felt the boys were more important, had more of a useful function . . . in terms of looking at futures, their futures were given a lot of thought, a lot of detail, a lot of advice, guidance, whereas the expectation for me was that it was not worth investing much, as I would just get married and have children and that was that.

As a result of Katherine having being placed in this role, the following sequence of events occurred when her mother became pregnant and too ill to look after Katherine's younger brother. Her caring role had been assigned to Katherine by virtue of her gender, with significant repercussions for Katherine's educational welfare which she had tried to ward off.

> *Katherine*: The expectation was I was the next eldest female so I was the carer and I would do this. I was staying on at school to do exams, but that was totally overlooked and no amount of persuading on my part would make my father see it differently. He'd made the decision.

Debbie's experience had also reflected the differential demands resulting from ascribed gender roles and her dislike of this.

> *Debbie*: My eldest brother is 52, my other brother is 48. I have two younger brothers in their twenties. We [her older sister and herself] were

left to bring them up. If I said I didn't have to get up in the night and said 'it's not my baby', I got a slap round the ear for that.

Even where women described having perceived their mother's needs as having overriding importance, their accounts revealed that they had still retained a capacity for self-expression and assertiveness throughout childhood. Frances described her relationship with her mother as follows:

Frances: My experience of loving from my mother was how much she needed me, how much she needed me to love her . . . I got affection and love for being a good girl, for taking care of her.

However, she also nominated her maternal grandfather as the other most important person in her childhood. She went on to describe how she had turned to him as a means of escape from her violent father. *Frances*: 'With my grandfather it was an escape route for me, a haven, because there was a lot of violence going on in my family . . . so I needed to get away from that, and I did with my grandad.' Winifred described having taken responsibility as a carer for her mother.

Winifred: As I say, my mother tended to be ill rather a lot. It used to worry me to death, I'm still conditioned to this now. Since I was about 12 I believed she was going to die imminently, and she used to pass out on me, not faint but go unconscious for some time. She got upset and passed out, you used to think, 'don't upset mother or she'll pass out', and God if she did pass out there was hell to pay.

Her parents subsequently forced Winifred to choose between her mother and her fiancé, employing the emotional blackmail that her mother would die if Winifred failed to break off their engagement. Winifred described the feeling of being responsible for her mother as persisting into adulthood; she also broke off her engagement. However, the fact of her becoming engaged, together with the distress she endured in breaking it off, 'It was terrible', indicated that however profound her own acceptance of her role as her mother's carer, she had still retained alternative desires.

Women's accounts also showed evidence of a capacity for assertiveness and self-expression in childhood in another way. Women may have kept their thoughts to themselves, but there were examples of them having had fierce feelings of injustice about their interests being disregarded, as opposed to them simply having accepted that their interests came second. In some cases they had vowed to take action to change the situation. The inhibiting factor seemed not to have lain in their own psyche, where such rebellious thoughts did not arise because the potential for them had been liquidated from the start. Instead it seemed to have lain in the hierarchical nature of the power relations between them and their parents which had constrained what they could do – with the threat or reality of physical assault possibly reinforcing adult dominance.

Jan: I was brought up in a fairly sort of standard attitude that if you misbehaved you were smacked. It was a fairly haphazard kind of justice. If my sister had started an argument with me, for example, and there was screaming and bawling and things, we'd both get slapped, because Mum would say, 'that means I've got the right one', irrespective of which one was actually causing the trouble. I used to feel those kinds of things were totally unjust.

Sue: I've suffered so much as a kid and in my teenage years, that I always used to think, 'When I grow up I won't have to do that, I won't have to eat cabbage.' I've been made to sit and eat cabbage, 'so I will – my grown up life must be happier.'

In theory, women could have been reading back on to childhood realizations which they had gained subsequently or through feminist therapy. However the content of their comments indicates that the feelings they refer to had come into being in childhood.

These findings therefore suggest that any explanatory account of young women's self-identity needs to register that they retain a capacity for assertiveness and self-expression. Rather than being seen as extinguished through the inegalitarian nature of current social relations, this capacity should be seen as being given little opportunity for expression in interpersonal interaction.

Relationships with fathers

Introduction

From women's accounts there also seemed to be at least as strong a case for interrogating the role of women's fathers in influencing their emotional wellbeing in childhood, as for focusing on women's interaction with their mothers (Sayers 1988). Women saw relationships with their fathers as having been important in their own right and as having a powerful effect on them. When asked who were the most important people as far as they were concerned when they were children, only three cited mothers as important, two of whom had no fathers and one whose father was violent. One woman, Ruth, commented that her father didn't figure very strongly in her childhood: 'He was very much married to his job – a very reserved man.' However she went on to indicate that the nature of the relationship had important repercussions for her. 'I missed the physical affection from my father that I saw other children getting and I felt very envious of them.' The majority of women cited their father and next 'parents' or in some cases 'grandparents' as the most important people to them while they were growing up. Women's perceptions of their relationships with their fathers in childhood also reflected the ways in which the gendered nature of social relations operated powerfully through father–daughter relationships.

Fathers as patriarchs – and perpetrators of abuse

There were several instances of women describing households in childhood being organized on the basis of fathers as ultimate authorities – with this role embodying the ideal of male supremacy. As this had happened, so it seemed to have contributed to eroding women's self-confidence as children. Debbie had been keen to find approval from her father, but he was hard to please. She described how he saw women as cooks and child bearers, second class citizens. Women of the family 'took a back seat'. *Sue* also saw her father as all powerful – 'I was always frightened of my father. He was a very Victorian sort of man. Very domineering . . .' As already discussed, Frances had had to seek escape routes from her father's violence.

Winifred was also one of two women in the sample whose relationship with their fathers had had a profoundly subordinating effect, through their fathers' sexual abuse of them. Her account brings out clearly the unequal power relationships involved.

> *Winifred*: It sounds so terribly bad but I felt I was his toy, his daughter, he thought the world of me but he didn't like me having boyfriends, one of the worst things was he made fun of my boyfriends, they were not made very welcome in the house, you know. Keep them standing on the doormat while I got ready . . . I realised as I grew older that he was aware I was a woman not a girl, sort of thing and he used to fondle my breasts which I hated . . . but I didn't – because I was so – didn't quite know how to say 'don't do that'.

Winifred's account also suggests how in a fairly common pattern, her father's abuse of her had been legitimated within family discourse, as resulting from his being denied the opportunity of alternative sexual expression.

> he and my mother were very different. She was . . . a very quiet retiring sensitive person, super sensitive actually, and I suspect my father was a much more physical sort of man. He wanted more physical love, this is what I felt.

> (Ward 1984: Ch. 5)

Gillian's account conveys the elements of insecurity, but also terror that sexual abuse can bring. Both her description of the abuse, and why it stopped, reveals how it had been rooted in her stepfather exercising his power over her.

Her description also indicates the way in which her stepfather's behaviour reflected the gendered assumption of men's sexual needs as pre-eminent (McLeod 1982).

> *Gillian*: When he started to abuse me . . . I remember the time I felt really scared was when my Mum was pregnant for the second time, and I know when she goes in hospital I'm going to be left there with him and I thought, 'What can I do?' I fought him most of the time, told him to get off, then to my relief my cousin came to stop with me. So he came nowhere near me at all.

Fathers as treasured companions

In contrast to such experiences, several of the women looking back saw their relationships with their fathers as very positive. They had been sources if not *the* source of profound emotional satisfaction. *Nina*: 'I've always felt and still do feel that I got everything that was good from my father. In terms of physical affection and emotional sustenance in the sense that . . . he accepted me as I was.' Olivia had always felt close to her father (more so than her mother). She had totally relied on him when at school. *Olivia*: 'He was very approachable, easy to talk to, we could agree to differ. There was nothing not loving, at the time.' *Irene*: 'I feel I got a lot of positive things from my father. He was just a very accepting, peace loving and tolerant sort of man. Within our relationship there were qualities which he showed me which I was then able to take on board.'

The women also described their fathers as having enhanced their creativity and their intellect and broadened their horizons. Their accounts conveyed the excitement of the 'window on the world' their fathers had offered. *Irene*: 'He would play with me, he was an artist and he would draw and make cardboard cut-outs of things and sit on the floor and play with me. And he wrote me stories . . . I'm just remembering a lot of fun with him.' Debbie's father in the early days was loving. *Debbie*: 'He would play. He would do DIY, making things. Making a car out of a box with a wheel on.' *Nina*: 'He encouraged me. Educated me and influenced my ideas and judgements because he was interested in many things, and it stuck.' *Mary*: 'He used to take me for walks. That's my image of him.' There were also echoes of these positive features in *Christine*'s account of her grandfather: 'I remember him as being the one who really catered to my imagination. He was the one who taught me the time. I used to go down to the library with him. I associate learning new things with him.'

This aspect of their father's behaviour had clearly been a great joy to the young women and they gained lasting benefit from it. It also gives the lie to the idea that fathers' behaviour is necessarily exploitative. However, men's participation as fathers in the more recreational forms of childcare with their daughters also raises questions about its gendered nature. It may reflect a situation where the organization of childcare is such as to continue to conserve for men some of the choicest forms of contact with children, as opposed to the drudgery of maintenance work which tends to be left to mothers (David and New 1985). Through a disproportionate share of the work of childcare still being placed on women in an uncollectivized, under-resourced way, it may be beyond women's individual energies, while still cast as an individual woman's responsibility (Popay 1992). Carrying out childcare in this way may also undermine the opportunities and energies women have to consider children's needs in depth (Hochschild 1990). It could go some way to explaining the lacklustre response from their mothers, which women in the sample had earlier complained of as failing to meet their emotional needs in childhood, e.g. 'always cross', physically undemonstrative – though 'into the role of feeding us'. It represents a terrible irony if, because of having to work too hard because of the present sexist division of labour in childcare, women can't meet what their children see as some of their most important needs.

The women's accounts of their father's and mother's respective roles also seemed to reflect the following gendered valuations being intertwined: a higher estimation of the value of public as opposed to domestic activity (Oakley 1976), greater tolerance of the demands that men's behaviour exacted because of the high status ascribed to men's work (Stacey and Price 1981: Ch. 3), and possibly higher valuation of men *per se*. For example, in Irene's account, her father's spasmodic appearances had in no way detracted from his importance to her.

Irene: He seemed to be someone who visited the house occasionally. He worked shifts, and he worked a very funny shift system, and I could never really get the hang of it. I never knew when he was going to be in, I always had to ask my mum if he was going to be in at night. But on those occasions when he did have time to spend with me I have got a lot of positive memories of that.

Mary had greatly valued her father, but when asked about the people who were important to her in childhood replied, 'not specially my Mum, she was just there.'

Louise: I suppose my dad was more important than my mother. He was a super man. He gave me a little extra – like music [crying]. He was a lovely man, very very kind, very nice [still crying] . . . I think in a way I was more attached to him than to my mother. My mother was always very good, went out of her way, always kind, looked after us very well physically, washing, cooking, as I grew up.

Women displayed some understanding of the difficulties that their mothers may have faced on an individual basis in meeting their needs as children.

Jan: When I think about my Mum and what she was able to do, I mean I feel quite defensive and protective towards her as a parent, because given the kind of situation she was having to work in, bringing up children on her own and having to work as well in badly paid jobs of one sort or another, she provided the best possible care that she could.

However, it was striking that despite the fact that all the women had had experience of feminist therapy, there was no reference in the group to feminist understandings about the structural position women occupy in relation to childcare.

Father's–mother's relationship: mother–daughter relationship

The women's accounts also reflected the powerful effect of the gendered nature of relationships in shaping their emotional wellbeing, as it operated through their father's relationship with their mother and influenced in turn their mother's relationship with them. The impact on mothers of the nature of their relationship with the young women's fathers, or the father's absence, could hold significant implications for how the young women's emotional needs fared. Jan's and Christine's poignant accounts brought out how women's primary role as childcarers, together with the dearth of resources preventing women from being comfortably self-sufficient as heads of households (Barrett and McIntosh 1982), and the stigmatized nature of this situation (Phoenix 1991), had suffused the experience of all concerned.

Jan: I became very self-sufficient emotionally, I don't remember ever really feeling I wanted or could expect to talk to her very much [her mother] about any particular problems or anything I might have because I think the main message I felt was she had enough to worry about – there she was on her own with these three daughters to bring up, terrible burden and things, and that it wasn't really possible to demand any more from her, than what she was already doing . . . because the thing about my dad was that he couldn't stand the responsibility of her being pregnant, and every time she was pregnant he would just disappear – which although he wasn't talked about much, those were the messages that we got.

Christine remembered her childhood as 'very secure, happy' nevertheless her father's rejection of her mother had had a formative influence on Christine's own emotional development.

Christine: My mother brought me up, I was an illegitimate child, my natural father was already married so my mother was still living with my grandparents and as a result of my birth we had to move to a different district of the city. I was brought up by my mother, grandmother and grandfather. My mother went back to work and was working full time, so the caretaking was very much shared between my grandmother and my mother and my grandfather . . . my grandmother was very much the dominant figure in terms of what I'd become as a personality as an adult – it's part very much of how my grandmother brought me up . . . the script my grandmother left me has been one I've probably been fighting against . . . 'never trust a man Christine, all men are bastards. Look what happened to your mother, your mother got deserted' . . . so that phrase really stuck in my mind and I resolved never ever to either sort of settle down with anybody or to get married.

Young women's comparative powerlessness as children

Introduction

The effects of the gendered nature of social relations on women's emotional wellbeing in childhood emerged as having been mediated in turn by another factor – women's comparative powerlessness as children. Recognition of children's position as an oppressed group within society, on the basis of their comparative powerlessness is one of the perspectives currently informing debates on childcare policy and practice. It has been particularly concerned with the way in which such comparative powerlessness is reflected in the limitations to children's legal rights (Fox Harding 1991), as in the difficulty children still have in 'divorcing' their parents or guardians if unhappy with their care (Cervi 1993). Nevertheless this standpoint also suggests that it is important to inspect adult–child relations generally, for manifestations of children's comparative powerlessness to the detriment of their well-being:

> The concept of oppression directs attention to fundamental social processes which are precise opposites to notions of value and respect, focusing on the myriad ways in which children are systematically seen as worthless, as lesser individuals or not really people in their own right
> (Ryan and Stubbs 1989: 226).

Such a perspective does not amount to crude 'adult-blaming'. It is concerned to tease out how the dimension of children's comparative powerlessness may run through social relations. For example, accounts of parenting in poverty have set out the sacrifices that parents may make for their children, to the extent of going without food and clothes themselves (Blackburn 1991). A focus on children's comparative powerlessness in relation to such a situation would also highlight the policy assumptions that disregard the material and care requirements of children – thereby presenting parents with daunting if not impossible tasks. It would consider the limitations to children's room for manoeuvre in such a situation and the consequences of this. It would also not assume that the effects of the adults' actions were benign from the child's standpoint. Therefore it would draw, where possible, on children's accounts to clarify the nature and significance of their experience for their welfare, as they saw it.

Applying such a perspective also has implications for the forms of intervention that are considered. For example, on the basis of analysing women's emotional wellbeing in terms of its gendered nature, Eichenbaum and Orbach argue for taking the primary burden of childcare off women individually and that it should be socialized and evenly divided between men and women. This is in the interests of the organization of childcare exercising a more egalitarian influence on women's emotional development (1985: Ch. 10). What Eichenbaum and Orbach do not consider in such a process is how work towards equalizing the power differential between adults and children may also need to be undertaken to secure more equitable conditions for women's development.

Factors mediating children's comparative powerlessness

A detailed exploration of the social circumstances of significant adults in women's lives in childhood was beyond this study's resources. Therefore extensive evidence on the characteristics of these circumstances which may have affected the adults' relationships with their children is lacking. Nevertheless, besides discussing some of the forms of dominating adult behaviour which had undermined their emotional wellbeing, women's accounts also indicated some of the ways in which it had been tempered and reinforced.

The presence or absence of other dimensions to inequality was implicated in the exercise of adult power. As has already been shown, young women's emotional wellbeing had been prey both to insidious and blatant sexism. As will be discussed, the impact of disablism, relative poverty and racism were also apparent.

From the women's accounts, adults had not consistently disregarded their interests in childhood. There was evidence of adults determinedly working with the young women's interests at heart. For example *Christine* typified the efforts of her grandmother, grandfather and mother on her behalf in childhood as, 'I was wrapped in cotton wool by all three of them.' Further work to unravel the factors militating in favour of adults' commitment to their children's wellbeing is therefore very important. Some of the complexity of what is involved in creating such commitment is revealed in Phoenix' study of teenage mothers. Against the stigmatizing approach to women in their teens becoming mothers, she found evidence of their deep commitment to the wellbeing of their children and in the harshest circumstances of material deprivation. The restricted options open to the women concerned, their desire for self-expression, female solidarity and social norms in their immediate circle, all played a part in creating such commitment. As Phoenix comments:

> Why were women who . . . might be expected to be engaging in youth cultural practices and developing 'style' . . . so content with motherhood? One reason is that most women interviewed had long anticipated that motherhood would be the most fulfilling aspect of their lives. The majority had expected that they would become mothers earlier rather than later . . . early motherhood was common in most women's social networks . . . In addition relatives, particularly mothers, were generally supportive in providing childcare and material resources . . . essential to the good outcomes found.
>
> (Phoenix 1991: 249–50)

Even where adults have children's interests at heart, it does not, of course, guarantee that children benefit. The power differential between the two parties means that the relationship may well not be equally on children's terms. This is revealed in *Nina*'s comment about her mother, 'I know, I suppose, intellectually that she probably did love us, but that was qualified because I couldn't actually feel it.'

There was also evidence from the women's accounts that despite the best of intents, adults' efforts on their children's behalf could be thwarted because of the social conditions adults themselves had been up against. In Christine's case, shortcomings in resources for women with disabilities to live independently and to care independently for their children (Morris 1991), came through as having limited her mother's efforts to care for Christine as her mother would have liked. Along with the gendered nature of Christine's mother's existence it had been a further tie that had bound her to *her* parent's household.

> *Christine*: I was protected from a lot of battles that went on between my mother and grandmother, I can just remember one occasion when I was eight, my mother wanted to leave home, and we were going to move to a bedsit, and I can remember sitting on the bed with my mother, she's a diabetic, and she was trying to explain to me that it would be very difficult to cope with me on my own as a diabetic, she was still having lots of comas at the time. And I think that's probably the most upsetting memory I've got as a child.

There was also evidence from the women's accounts that their own behaviour as children towards adults could be dominating. The evidence was scanty and interestingly enough came from a childhood relationship which the woman herself – Esther – identified as centred on her interests. *Esther*: 'I must have been quite a trial to my mother because I was so self-willed, argumentative, but I don't remember any come-back from that in our relationship.'

Despite pointing to various ways in which adult power was mediated, women's accounts still indicated that in its own right it had been a threat to their emotional wellbeing in childhood.

The undermining effect of children's comparative powerlessness

Women's accounts centred on their interactions with parents or parent figures but indicated that the effects of children's comparative powerlessness permeated social relationships more generally. For example, Gillian had been taken into care and removed from home for her protection after her stepfather's abuse of her. Nevertheless it had been Gillian who was removed from home, rather than measures being taken for the removal of the stepfather. As Hudson has commented 'great ambivalence still remains about using the criminal law as a mechanism for dealing with child sexual abuse' (1992: Ch. 7).

In relation to interactions with their parents and parent figures, women's accounts brought out how their comparative powerlessness as children had had the following effects. It had meant that the power to ensure that their emotional needs as children were met, had lain with the adults concerned. There was also evidence of sexual and physical abuse and that adults had tended to set the terms on which affection was offered. There was evidence of a lack of recognition of the value of the emotional resources and caring young women had offered as children. Finally, there was evidence of exclusion from adult discourse and of young women's complaints as children not being heard. These dimensions to young women's experience in childhood are discussed in turn.

Family networks as sites of adult power

Almost without exception, the people women identified as the most important to them as they had been growing up were within the immediate networks of their family of origin. The two exceptions concerned women who had undertaken a good deal of their care, although the status of a family member – 'substitute mother' had even been conferred on one of these. Otherwise, parents, grandparents, siblings, sometimes an aunt or uncle were named. Relationships with siblings could be of significance for women's emotional wellbeing. They could be the source of demands on young women to care, such as in Debbie's and Katherine's case, which could lead to their own needs being undermined. They could provide affection and opportunities for solidarity *vis-à-vis* adults, as *Debbie* described having been the case in her relationship with her sister: 'two peas outside the pod'. They could also provide opportunities for rivalry or domination. *Esther*: 'I've got a brother, we were quite close when we were young. But as we got older there was quite a lot of jealously, he was jealous of me because I went to grammar school, I was really quite bossy.'

Nevertheless, one or more adult parent figures in family networks consistently emerged as most influential in determining whether young women's need for affection had been met in childhood or whether the affection and caring young women offered had been valued. That the initiative for young women's emotional needs being met or not in relationships with adult parent figures had lain with the adults, was implied in accounts of positive experiences.

> *Beatrice*: I can't think of anything as a child which would have been bad. The sort of worries I would have as a child were if I got home from school at lunchtime and Mum wasn't in . . . She was at a neighbours.

> *Esther*: I had a very happy childhood . . . we weren't well off, Mum died about two years ago. I loved my mum . . . We used to go to the Bull Ring quite a lot, me and my mum, and we'd have winkles. Sucking on crab claws great . . . People you live with as a child must have an effect . . . my parents influenced who I am. I just think they gave me a really good beginning in life.

That the initiatives for young women's emotional needs being met had lain with adults was also implied where women had had *some* concerns about their emotional needs being met. Mary, for instance, commented that her aunt and father had conveyed the idea that her actions always needed their approval. *Mary*: 'I still need approval, that's becoming less now I'm becoming more established but, I still do need it.' Tina did not elaborate on her concerns but commented that she had come to realize that her family had been somewhat old-fashioned in terms of seeking to control and direct their children's behaviour. Annie identified 'a certain lack of confidence' stemming from the fact that her mother had been disappointed in her because she hadn't shared certain aptitudes her mother had had. From contact with her neighbour who was an 'honorary mother' Annie felt she had gained confidence because of the neighbour's emphasis on women's self-fulfilment. *Annie*: 'It made me feel free to do what I wanted to do, instead of doing what I was expected to do.'

The proof that the initiative for young women's emotional needs being met or not in relationships with adult parent figures had lain with the adults, came from women's accounts of when those relationships had failed to meet their emotional needs. For then, although young women had done what they could, the power to reverse the situation had not been theirs to command.

> *Gillian*: My childhood was terrible, really bad. From the age of six my stepdad used to find an excuse to smack me . . . I couldn't get my mother to stop him. When I was 11 or 12 my stepdad started to abuse me and always told me not to tell my mum, and I didn't because when I did want to tell her I knew she wouldn't believe me. It got so bad I ran away from home, then the truth came out. I told my auntie about it, my uncle believed me but my mum still didn't believe me, I still wonder why she wouldn't . . . My stepdad always made out to her I was a liar. So the most important person in my life was me. I couldn't trust anybody, couldn't feel for anybody.

While spared the experience of physical violence, Ruth's and Zoë's accounts reflected the same adult–child power relations in operation.

> *Zoë*: The most loving relationship I had was with my father who died when I was 12. My mother . . . I wouldn't say she was overtly loving . . . but I had found it was quite easy to have a cosy loving relationship with my father . . . I always had a pet dog and I found a lot of solace in the dog. A lot of people put their love onto the dog.

Besides getting little affection from her father, Ruth also described getting little from her mother.

> *Ruth*: My mother is a very dominant woman, really. She came from a background where displays of affection were considered unnecessary. So I gained my affection from others by being creative, really. I used to write funny stories for others and illustrate them, for my friends and my brothers.

Sexual abuse and physical assault

The gendered nature of the childhood sexual abuse suffered by two women in our sample has already been referred to. It has also been argued (Kelly 1988) that such abuse reflects ageist assumptions by perpetrators, of children's comparative vulnerability. Among the sample there were accounts of physical assault too. Gillian described experiencing a severe degree of brutality.

> *Gillian*: My stepdad used to use my face as a football. The amount of times I went to hospital he fractured my face this side, it was really bad, I had to have 24 X-rays. I was put in a home for nine months and those

nine months were Heaven. I never felt so good in all my life because I was away from the family.

Other women reported less severe assaults but still with undermining effects. Debbie described how after her father had slapped her, she had checked herself voicing her thoughts to her father about how unfair it was that she had to get up in the night to look after her younger brother. *Debbie*: 'At fifteen if you feel you'll be subjected to physical violence, you keep your mouth shut next time.' Debbie's account fits the pattern of evidence that physical violence is routinely used in the home (Newson and Newson 1976) to assert adult authority over children.

Sue also described how in her experience, growing up had been characterized by a psychological climate of fear, instituted as a result of adult authority.

> *Sue*: I was frightened when I was growing up. My mother died, and he [her father] wouldn't let me grow up. Wouldn't let me wear makeup, things like that . . . Betty my stepmother said he could be very loving. I saw he could be really horrid . . . What I remember most about childhood is dreading going home. When I was at school I used to get a later train and put off going home.

Young women's need for affection met on adult terms

Instances of sexual abuse and physical assault could be seen as stark examples of adult behaviour undermining children's emotional wellbeing. However, women's accounts suggested that these should be placed in the context of evidence that more generally their need for affection had tended to be met on adults' terms. This tendency may have reflected pressures parents were under as adults. For example, the scantiness of attention beyond basic caretaking, complained of in women's accounts, could be seen as having reflected the overwhelming nature of their mother's gendered responsibilities. Though not a source of complaint for the most part from women in our sample, attention from fathers had had to be fitted in with employment routines. Nevertheless, evidence of the damage that could ensue through children's need for affection being met on adult terms is provided respectively by Zoë's and Sue's experience and Gillian's with her own father. Zoë's account reflected what has been identified as a continuing tendency on adults' part to underestimate the profound nature of children's feelings following bereavement (Wallbank 1992). Zoë described how in the pressures on her mother to keep the family going after Zoë's father's death, Zoë's need to grieve had got scant recognition.

> *Zoë*: My mum had to be very independent and supportive and did the right thing by us and she kept the house and went back to college and did

some O levels and started teaching and she did all the right things . . . being twelve at the time [father] died I was a nonentity really, I was just quiet and that was it and nobody was at all concerned at how I was feeling, they just thought I was OK. I didn't even try and seek affection and love from her [her mother].

Sue described how her relationship with her stepmother had not provided compensation for the climate of fear her father had produced as she grew up. Instead, Sue had felt that her needs counted for little – that she was an intruder in her own family.

Sue: She's [her stepmother] not naturally a motherly person, she would hand you a towel round the door and run off, if you were sick. Basically a very selfish person, really couldn't cope with me I suppose. I've always felt in the way. Whether I was a threat to her relationship with my father or what I don't know. I spent all my teenage years feeling in the way.

After Gillian's maltreatment by her stepfather she had been desperate for some contact with her own father and affection from him, but from her faltering account – half excusing him – what she had got had been very sparse, ensuring that she disrupted his life to a minimum.

Gillian: When I think about it now, I was pushing myself on to him. I'd phone him up, go down, but I kept thinking to myself, he wasn't showing me no love either. He was just a man, there, then I found out he'd got married, and I'd got a halfbrother . . . my dad asked me about how I was getting on at school but that was it. I don't think we could talk much. He was the quiet type. I suppose because he was always working, when he came in he was tired and all he wanted to do was have his dinner and go down the pub with his friends. He didn't go out much, only now and again, just to have a drink, or his friends would come round.

Lack of recognition for affection and caring offered to adults

Women's accounts indicated that adult–child hierarchies could also result in lack of recognition for the affection and caring they had offered to adults, as well as limitations to the affection they had received. For example, neither Winifred, Debbie nor Katherine had gained a sense of esteem from their extensive efforts at caring. Instead it had been viewed as their duty and they had courted punishment if they had jibbed at what they were expected to do, or fell below adult standards in any way. Their experience here could be seen as a microcosm of young carers' experience generally, in that their efforts are only just beginning to gain recognition (Aldridge and Becker 1993). Jan also described how she had become very 'self-sufficient' emotionally because she had felt she could not make demands on her mother as she was so overburdened with looking after three daughters on her own. However, she had had no sense of acknowledgement of her self-restraint, nor the demands it made on her to exercise it. The frustration and despondency young women could experience as their heart-felt efforts received little recognition from parents comes through in Frances' and Debbie's comments: *Frances*: 'They [parents] have high expectations of you but tend not to praise the good. Just take it for granted . . . I mean in later years they say they were proud of you, but not at the time.'

Debbie: They keep changing the rules. You can't get in. You do what they [parents] want. You've completed the task and can enter the circle. Then they say, 'ah, but' . . . so you're always trying to achieve the impossible.

Exclusion from adult discourse

Young women also identified how they had often been excluded from adult discourse within family networks. The result was to leave their emotional needs unaddressed. Katherine described how she had been allowed to participate in the physical caretaking of a major life event, but had not been allowed entry into the spoken and shared understandings which would have represented at least token equality at this time between parent and child.

Katherine: But then my mother got pregnant when I was eight or nine and lost the baby . . . I remember her going into hospital to have the baby, they'd all been excited about it, then my father coming home one night and I'd got to help him put all the baby things away and we'd got to hide them or move them out. So I helped him with this, so I gathered the baby wasn't coming home. When she [her mother] came out she was obviously really upset but it was never spoken about, it wasn't shared.

Gillian described how even the true nature of her parentage had been kept from her for many years by her own mother. It meant that across early childhood she had thought she had no other option as a father than her stepfather who was abusing her.

Gillian: My stepdad used to find an excuse to smack me – at the age of seven I found out why he wasn't my real dad. When I was at school Mom phoned up, and when I came back I said, 'Who's this' And she said, 'Your dad'. And I thought *he* was my dad.

Sue's peripheral position is illustrated in how she had found out *by chance* her father was remarrying, after the traumatic death of her mother in a car accident several years earlier. The shock of finding out in this way is conveyed in how the details of the scene of the revelation are etched in her memory.

> *Sue*: My mother died when I was nine, I never got on well with my father, I felt – I was very close to my mother. And then she died when I was nine . . . I then muddled on with my father till I was 13, he got married again then. He didn't tell me, I found out from a lady at the bus stop, a local farmer, they bought the eggs from there, he was getting married on October 27, and I didn't know.

Unheard complaints

The extensive injuries Gillian sustained did eventually bring her to the attention of the childcare authorities. Otherwise, a lack of attention in childhood to women's accounts of injustice experienced then could be seen as representing a further dimension to their comparative powerlessness as children which had undermined their emotional wellbeing. Their accounts were only destined to receive serious attention as reflecting matters requiring remedying, in adulthood, through feminist therapy. Then of course, they received attention as regards the possible after-effects of childhood experience on the women as adults.

Bearing in mind the age range of the women in the sample – with childhoods coming to an end about ten years previously – it could be argued that since that time there have been positive changes in the amount of attention and the credibility given to children's accounts of maltreatment by adults. For example, work to document and give recognition to children's accounts of sexual and physical abuse is now an integral part of childcare practice in social work (Frost 1992). Confidential telephone lines have been set up specifically to provide children with an opportunity to give their accounts and seek help (Fox Harding 1991: 194). There has also been use of the media and publications for children, drawing on other children's experiences to encourage them not to feel isolated but more confident in speaking out (Bain and Sanders 1990).

Despite these developments, commentators such as Valentine (1989) have argued that much of what *children* define as abusive behaviour by adults may go unaddressed because it is routine, universal and neither recognized as abuse nor taken up by the childcare system. She argues that damage to a child's welfare may not necessarily be brought about by the onset of actual physical or sexual abuse. Instead, the child's morale may be profoundly undermined in routine ways. Speaking of the children she interviewed she writes

> Abuse for the child (by adults) was also experienced as a state of being – it was not just an event definable by a set of incidents. It thus covered

manipulation, misunderstanding, invalidating, indifference, lies, mystification, abandonment. Viewed in this way all children, whether in care or not, experienced these to some degree.

(Valentine 1989: 134)

Valentine's findings suggest that the legitimation of children's accounts of the state of their emotional wellbeing may still have far to go; and as such reflects the pervasive nature of adult–child unequal power relations.

The role of feminist therapy in recall

Two of the women in our study, Irene and Jan, described becoming aware for the first time during feminist therapy of certain dimensions to their childhood experience which they had previously forgotten.

> *Irene*: What I would have told you before I started coming here is really very different to how I see it now . . . how I did see it was I had a very close relationship as a young child, I felt I had a lot of physical affection . . . I can now recollect things that were said to me – very early in childhood and remembering that things were not right, things were said to me that were really quite cruel. She [her mother] meant them that way and she had her own reasons for saying these things. And that those things have affected me quite badly and it's only now that I'm realizing how awful it was, and how – I mean I don't think she ever accepted me for what I was.

Jan described how before coming to the feminist therapy centre she could never remember being upset by her father's behaviour when she was a child. However, since coming, she realized that previously she had not allowed herself to be upset.

> *Jan*: I can remember feeling all the various things I've said I felt, angry with my father, that I wasn't getting the things other children had, but I couldn't remember crying about it. I actually cried for the first time at the therapy centre which took me by surprise I think really, because I hadn't let myself feel upset about it at all.

Several responses are possible to these accounts. First, scepticism, that what is being described is the power of suggestion on the counsellor's part distorting memories. Against this, once the women themselves had recall, they clearly thought that the memories fitted their experience. The memories also made aspects of their experience which had previously puzzled them understandable – such as the depths of the distress which they had undergone since childhood. Another response is that because it was so painful for women in childhood to face what was being done to them, they had suppressed their feelings at the time and totally repressed the memory of what had happened. As Miller writes,

When vital needs are frustrated and children are instead abused for the sake of adults' needs . . . The normal reactions to such injury should be anger and pain; since children in this hurtful kind of environment, however, are forbidden to express their anger and since it would be unbearable to experience their pain all alone, they are compelled to suppress their feelings, repress all memory of the trauma, and idealise those guilty of the abuse. Later they will have *no memory of what was done to them* (author's emphasis).

(Miller 1989: 144)

The problem with this analysis is that not all abusive behaviour on adult's part is expunged from children's memory, nor are the adults idealized – as is exemplified in Gillian's account of her experience. A third response is that whatever the exact mechanisms of memory at work, it is possible to retrieve the most unpleasant and frightening memories which may have been 'lost' – when feeling supported and encouraged to do so. This is exemplified in the practice of Crawford, Kippax, Onyx, et al., who fostered groups where members encouraged each other to recall and analyse the social significance of emotionally charged memories. They found

in the context of studying emotion, we must cope with the commonsense idea that experiences associated with strong negative emotions will be irretrievably forgotten. We have not found this. . . . Many of our memories and those of students and others who have given us memories, included experiences involving shame, guilt, revulsion. It is possible to retrieve, reflect upon and reinterpret material long forgotten, at any stage of our lives.

(Crawford, Kippax, Onyx, et al. 1992: 166)

On these grounds, Jan and Irene's recall may stem from finding, in their contact with the feminist therapy centre in question, an environment where their emotional wellbeing was accorded prime importance as was the opportunity to give their account of it (see Chapter 5). In this case the role of feminist therapy in recall may emerge, not as producing distortion, but facilitating clarity through providing resources which may still be in short supply to children in childhood, as a reflection of their comparative powerlessness *vis-à-vis* adults.

The impact of other social divisions on women's emotional wellbeing in childhood

In women's accounts, the influence of the gendered nature of social relations on women's emotional wellbeing in childhood therefore emerged as having been mediated by children's comparative powerlessness. However, the effects of gender and children's comparative powerlessness had, in turn, been mediated by other social divisions.

Jan's account brought out the undermining effects of the experience of relative poverty. Her mother, being unable to indulge in conspicuous consumption in a consumerist society, had left Jan feeling materially deprived.

> *Jan*: In terms of my mother being able to show us the kind of attention other children had, say at Christmas, when it came to being able to give really big lavish presents, I mean she couldn't do that. That's what I'm most aware of as a child . . . we were actually relatively poorly off. And resenting that very much.

Jan also commented on how she had come to see that the expectation that children would not participate in adult discourse, 'There was this big division between children and adults.' – a situation which had compounded her emotional isolation – might have been a facet of her class position.

> *Jan*: Later on I had a friend when I was about 14, who came from quite a middle-class family, who had obviously got more liberal attitudes towards bringing up their children, so the way she related to adults I remember noticing was very different to how I did. Although she was 14, and I was 14 as well, she would talk to adults on a very much one-to-one basis and could demand the same kind of listening and respect . . . while I would never expect to be able to talk to adults like that at all.

In Irene's case, she had come to acknowledge how the disablist nature of social relations had shaped her mother's reactions to her with adverse effects. Irene described how at the core of her mother's lack of acceptance of her lay her mother's response to her disability – that Irene was somehow inferior because of it (see Morris 1991: Chs. 2 and 3). Moreover, Irene had also felt trapped in a double bind. She had felt under pressure to treat her disability as a taboo subject, to deny it being part of her experience. In that way the possibility of exploring its positive aspects had been closed off from her.

> After I was born and while I was still in hospital I contracted osteo-arthritis, and ended up having one arm shorter than the other, so I have only limited mobility in my shoulder. I mean in effect it doesn't really have much effect on my life, but I know that she [her mother] was quite psychologically ill for a couple of years, not seriously ill, I just don't feel she could ever accept me the way I was. I should have been perfect and I think she felt it was her fault. And because of that I got a lot of underlying messages that it wasn't OK for me to admit I had any

particular feelings about what had happened to me, I had to keep all those hidden. And that was really quite disastrous.

(Morris 1991: Ch. 1)

Gillian did not specify her experience of abuse as having been mediated by racism. However, she described a shift in the balance of power relations when her brothers had arrived. This suggested that she and her mother had also been battling with what Ahmed has referred to as the vulnerability that 'incomplete and divided families' resulting from the structural problems of Third World migration can produce (Ahmed 1986: 153). This had been in addition to the sexist and ageist nature of Gillian's stepfather's behaviour.

Gillian: My two brothers stepped in then. They wasn't living with us before, they were in Jamaica, and they came when I was 14. I could only go out when they went out and came back when they came in. It was all right because I got out, and when I got out I could do what I wanted, then come home with my brothers.

Legacy for future wellbeing?

Introduction

Women's accounts of primary relationships in childhood therefore indicated that they had been a medium through which the interplay of a range of social inequalities had affected their emotional wellbeing. Although not uniformly so, the consequences could also be profoundly undermining. The remaining question to consider is in what ways if any, women's accounts suggested that the effects of childhood experience had continued to influence their emotional wellbeing. The crucial issue emerged as being the extent to which the following needs on young women's part had been met in childhood: both their need for affection, and for the affection and care they offered, to be valued.

A relatively positive legacy

Where women either did not suggest such needs had failed to be met, or had only failed to be met to a minor degree, they described feeling relatively free to pursue their own interests in subsequent relationships in adulthood. Beatrice who had identified nothing as 'being bad' in childhood saw no major undermining effects accruing from childhood experience. Esther described her childhood as amounting to 'a really good beginning to my life'. Louise described 'nothing standing out as unloving or uncaring' and love of music as being the chief influence in her life that had carried forward.

Annie, Mary and Tina, for example, only identified minor stumbling blocks in their approach to relationships in adult life, arising as a result of minor shortcomings in childhood relationships (see page 42). In Annie's case this amounted to a degree of lack of confidence, in Mary's a greater need for approval than she thought was objectively necessary, in Tina's some lingering sense that the influence of comparatively elderly parents had resulted in her having some 'old fashioned ideas'. Christine's experience was mixed. She described receiving a wealth of affection in childhood. However, she also described her grandmother's attempt to set the terms on which Christine would give affection to men in future as subsequently inhibiting.

> *Christine*: I think the script my grandmother left me – 'never trust a man' – carried forward through most of my twenties . . . I was always the first to leave relationships. I could never be the one who was left. I always made sure I got out first.

These scenarios suggest caution in seeing women's emotional distress in adulthood as necessarily arising from childhood.

A negative legacy from childhood

However, there were a substantial number of women who described themselves as having experienced a marked absence of affection in childhood, together with their attempts at offering care and affection being discouraged. This had not annihilated their capacity for assertiveness and self-expression, but had resulted in their acquiring negative frames of reference in relation to themselves and their interaction with other people. These took a variety of forms but the following seemed to be the main tendencies: feeling little right to affection or happiness; a low sense of self-worth; being inclined to take a subordinate position in relationships, feeling scared to pursue love as an adult.

These tendencies are set out in turn. However, it is important to note that even where the women concerned had commented on having had one parent or parent-figure who had offered loving acceptance – as in the case of Nina, Olivia and Irene – it had not necessarily neutralized these effects. *Nina* described how she felt her profound lack of self-confidence went back 'to being raised as being not capable somehow'. She felt sure it had had an effect on her as she grew up, saying, 'I think I've spent a lot of time with my mother looking over my shoulder.' *Olivia* had always felt that there has been nothing 'not loving' about her relationship with her father. Nevertheless this still did not seem to counterbalance the lack of self-worth she felt she had acquired in childhood, which she had come to feel was implicated in subsequently developing bulimia. She described how her day-to-day care had been very much in her mother's hands. Throughout her childhood she had never felt accepted on a par with her brother by her mother – whatever she had tried to do to get her affection.

Sue, Debbie and Zoë described how in different ways they had come to feel they had little right to affection or happiness.

> *Sue*: I've had to cope with everything myself, a very lonely sort of existence . . . I think that's why I've lived on my own so long now. It's become my life position . . . consciously I see that a man living in my home . . . it's going to be like it was with my dad.

Through her childhood, *Zoë* came to feel that it was the norm for her not to feel happy. 'It was never an expectation that I should be happy. I was really quite happy to be, A, on my own and, B, not happy. I didn't really expect anything else because that was my experience.'

Ruth and Katherine both described ways in which their relationship with their parents – one now dead – still left them feeling that they had yet to demonstrate their personal worth.

> *Katherine*: I felt I had to show my father I did have potential, and when he died, I knew I hadn't reached it, and still haven't, I was so angry with him for dying . . . I'm left with that, and still ambitious, still pushing myself, still seeking potential.

Ruth described her mother as having been unable to accept any personal weakness on Ruth's part and spoke of the 'wasted years' of her life.

> *Ruth*: wasted because I didn't have enough self-esteem. I grew up with the idea there were things I *had* to be good at. I've always tended to have a low opinion of myself and the sad part of it is, that what I have to offer belies this silly idea of low self-esteem. You see other people who have half as much ability, but a lot of self confidence.

The original impact on Irene of a similar form of interaction continued to reverberate years later in her career.

> *Irene*: This isn't the first time I've given up a job, because I didn't feel I could cope, but . . . on both occasions I've been told they don't know what I'm worrying about, my work is perfectly adequate, 'You're very good at it', but that isn't how it seems to me. It feels like I should be doing something more, or I should be doing something perfectly, that's the message I got from my mother . . . you know, you've got to be perfect, but you're not . . . and you never will be. And it's been like banging my head against a brick wall.

Both Irene and Jan also described how the devaluing of their capacity to give and receive affection had exposed them to the tendency to take a subordinate position in subsequent relationships.

Jan: Being brought up in the way I was . . . I wasn't taught anything about what I might want for myself out of a relationship . . . you've got low sights, you didn't really expect very much, you didn't . . . get very much emotional or physical satisfaction.

Winifred also described how in her childhood her parents' tendency to subordinate her need for affection and their devaluation of what she offered, by subjecting it to unrealistic tests, had contributed to her feeling throughout adulthood – though with some resentment – that her main aim should be to put other people's needs first in relationships. 'I've been super-accountable.'

Finally, the frightening nature of some of the women's childhood experiences had left them scared to pursue love as an adult. Frances described how she had sought as a child to build a loving relationship with her grandfather as a safe alternative to the destructive effect of her father's violence. In the process of doing so (as she had later come to perceive through contact with the Women's Therapy Centre), she had got stuck with the idea that it was this type of relationship that would guarantee a safe experience of love. So she had sought to reproduce it even when it might not have been appropriate to her other needs.

Frances: It kept me going, my grandad, . . . but every time I'd get a bit shaky in my life then I'd try and set that relationship up with somebody. It made me feel safe, and that's what I managed to do in fact. But the point was it restricted my growth as well, kind of – that was an OK relationship for a child but it's not an OK relationship for an adult.

Gillian's fears of loving, resulting from her experience of abuse in childhood took a more direct form. She talked at length about how she felt her relationship with her stepfather affected her in adult life, that she was

not able to love the way I want to . . . I'm scared to love. Scared of saying and doing the wrong things. Scared to get involved seriously . . . not able to give someone the opportunity to really know me. Grant is the only person I've let into my secret life.

It is not being argued that these frames of reference left by the women's childhood experience determined the course of women's emotional wellbeing in adult life. However, their nature suggests that they might put the women concerned at a disadvantage in pursuing their own interests through relationships.

Conclusions

Women's accounts of primary personal relationships in childhood point to the limitations of depicting the state of women's emotional wellbeing as one of psychological passivity accruing from subordination through gender, primarily mediated by the mother–daughter relationship. There is evidence of young women's capacity for assertiveness and self-expression being retained, although it can be severely circumscribed. Direct and indirect relationships with fathers also emerge as significant. The impact of a range of social inequalities, including children's comparative powerlessness in interaction with gender is apparent. The consequences of childhood experience do not seem to be uniformly undermining for women's subsequent self-esteem. However, when they are so to a profound degree, not only has young women's need to receive affection in childhood been grossly undervalued – as pinpointed in existing literature on feminist therapy – but also their capacity to give affection.

three

Having a relationship:
women's emotional wellbeing
in adult relationships

Introduction

Women cited a range of personal relationships as being of primary importance in their adult lives: heterosexual and lesbian relationships, their relationships with their children and parents, female friendships and occasionally friendships with men. The significance of the tenor of these relationships for women's emotional wellbeing is analysed in turn.

This reveals the importance of the gendered nature of these relationships, but also the importance of the impact of other social divisions. For example, the interplay of heterosexism and children's comparative powerlessness comes into focus. As this happens, it also becomes clear that the legacy of subordination in childhood does not alone determine the state of women's emotional equilibrium in adulthood.

The role of the interaction of multiple social divisions in contributing to women's emotional wellbeing also emerges as important in other ways. Within what otherwise tend to be hierarchically structured relationships such as gendered heterosexual relations, a male partner can also behave in an equitable or supportive way. There is also some evidence of women behaving in a dominating way. Where parties to a relationship occupy a position of apparent equivalence, e.g. in the case of friendships with other women and lesbian relationships, the tendency is for these relationships to offer better opportunities for the emotional needs of both to be met in a mutually satisfying way. Nevertheless, such equivalence does not offer a guarantee of freedom from the experience of domination and subordination in relationships. Where fuller evidence is available, it indicates that explaining these apparent contradictions needs to draw on the possibility of other social divisions being in play.

The fluid nature of the impact of social inequalities on women's emotional wellbeing is illustrated by evidence that women's emotional identity cannot be characterized as solely consisting of a subordinate psyche – always putting others needs first. There is evidence of a tendency on the part of women in our study to subordinate behaviour, but their accounts also consistently demonstrate a capacity for self-expression and assertiveness and the receipt of affection. This capacity is either nourished by comparatively egalitarian relationships which give it a chance to flower, or undermined by hierarchical relationships in which women are the subordinate party, or it can become superseded by dominating behaviour as women become the dominant party.

Heterosexual relationships

Their gendered nature

With one exception (Tina) all the women nominated one or more heterosexual relationships as among the most important in their adult life. Their gendered nature emerged in a number of ways. Several women gave graphic accounts of how in entering such relationships they had been conditioned by what they now recognized to be general ideological pressures. These were to accept the idea that their personal worth and identity lay in heterosexual relationships or marriage designed to service men's needs (Hemmings 1982, Sarsby 1983).

> *Ruth*: There was a run of not very important relationships with men . . . really perhaps I shouldn't say this, but I think it's true for many women, this idea you have to be married to be socially acceptable and all the rest of it. I regret very much. But I wasn't mature enough, and perhaps the women's movement wasn't mature enough to make me feel enough of a woman in my own right.

> *Zoë*: In previous relationships I've just lost myself in the relationship and wanted that to be the perfect entity . . . the myth of the perfect relationship . . . When I first met him [current partner] I was doing the same. It's been as the relationship deteriorated that I've got myself back again.

> *Jan*: I think that's one of the contradictory things about being a girl – that I wasn't taught anything about what I might want for myself out of a relationship, it was all very much in the terms of 'don't get boys excited'. I mean you've got low sights, you didn't really expect very much, you didn't sort of get very much emotional or physical satisfaction.

In keeping with Raymond's analysis (1986), women's accounts also indicated that women enacting the role of emotional carers could provide a major mechanism for enshrining the existence of male dominance and ensuring its continuation. As illustrated in Nina and Sue's accounts, this took the form of the burden of servicing and maintaining relationships being on women's shoulders through such means as tuning their activities to male needs; ensuring that men were not overburdened by *their* demands; and accepting responsibility for avoiding the failure of the relationship.

> *Nina*: I think I came into marriage with an idea of how life should be, and how I should behave, and took on a lot of responsibility for making the marriage work much more than I should, to the extent of suppressing a large part of myself. I suppressed the need for contact with other people, different sexual outlets. I was modelling myself to his image of you know, how he would like me to be, you know 'my image of his image' as it were. I don't think that was in any way realistic.

Sue's account of her second major heterosexual relationship indicated the lengths she was prepared to go to maintain it, despite her experience of her first relationship as domineering.

> *Sue*: with Gary . . . I was prepared to adapt my life to the life he wanted to lead, going to the caravan site, etc. And also it was hard work emotionally, with his wife leaving him, he feels he can't hang on to women . . . he could be hard work in some respects, you've got to boost him, like 'You're wonderful'.

Women's psychological subordination as an explanation

Superficially, women's accounts of enacting the gendered role of emotional carers in a way that subordinated their interests also confirmed a central thesis in writings informing feminist therapy. This is that through their gendered childhood development, women introject the identity of a carer, so that placing others' needs first to the detriment of their own becomes, emotionally-speaking, women's first nature (see Chapter 1). However, a fuller account of the experience of heterosexual relationships on the part of the women in our study demonstrates that the state of women's emotional wellbeing cannot be framed solely in terms of women's psychological subordination. For example, although the women concerned – as in the case of Sue and Nina – might have devoted an enormous amount of energy and commitment to serving men's emotional needs, they could come to resent the situation they were in. Both Sue and Nina, before engaging in feminist therapy, had left their respective male partners. Women's accounts also demonstrated that, at times, the onset of heterosexual relationships could represent assertive, self-expressive behaviour on their part.

> *Christine*: I think basically I tend to pick men in whom I recognize female attributes and that leads me on to my husband . . . I found him

very female, physically he was softer, and the characteristics or attributes he'd got – the non-violence, more female.

Winifred: I met my husband again, funnily enough not only did I love him but I liked him. I'd never met anybody I particularly liked so I thought it was a good basis for a marriage.

The fate of women's emotional wellbeing in such relationships also cannot be discussed in terms of their attributes and actions alone. Their male partners' role has to be considered

Male partners' sexist behaviour

Women's room for manoeuvre in obtaining emotional fulfilment in their heterosexual relationships emerged as being circumscribed to a considerable extent by men's sexist behaviour in its own right. Norwood has popularized the idea that 'women love too much', i.e. that women's unhappiness in heterosexual relationships stems from their addiction to loving men, irrespective of the damaging effect of the men's behaviour on their emotional wellbeing (1986, 1988). However, as Andrews (1989) has pointed out, failure to incorporate the dimension of men's behaviour in its own right into this analysis, risks exempting men's behaviour from criticism. It also risks ascribing too much responsibility for the tenor of heterosexual relationships to women, pathologizing their behaviour in the process and possibly contributing to undermining women's self-esteem further.

The predominant tendency in women's accounts of their experience was for heterosexual relationships to be conducted by men 'on their own terms' giving preeminence to their emotional needs. Christine described how her husband did not share her commitment to serial monogamy but felt other sexual relationships were needed outside the central relationship, acted accordingly, and would not move on this point.

Christine: I lay awake at night when he was out, feeling absolutely desperate. And I think at that stage I would take anything to block it out. Tranquillisers, you name it I just knocked myself out . . . I thought, 'I just can't cope with this game playing that's going on.' I was being really wound up, so I left. I couldn't resolve my feelings about it and six months later he was still in contact through work. I went back on his terms.

In Winifred's case the medium through which her husband expressed his disregard of her emotional needs was not sexual behaviour, but long-term denial of the importance of her ambitions and the draining effect on her of care for their child with learning difficulties.

Winifred: I've always tried desperately to have a career . . . all along my married life . . . he's [her husband] never given any credence to it, not important. If I said 'I've got a job' he'd say 'Great, but don't let it make any difference to us' . . . I feel what I've missed in marriage is at the bad times, I've wanted someone to hold my hand. The other day we had a row over Kim and he said, 'You're a grown woman you ought to be able to stand up on your own feet.' If I cried he'd go. He doesn't like emotions.

A further way in which relationships tended to be conducted on men's terms was through pressure on women to lose their own identity to fit in with men's ideas or interests. Sue described the first man she had lived with after leaving home as 'very very nice', but then went on to describe the following feature of their relationship. *Sue*: 'I'd gone from my father who was very domineering to Tony who in some ways held me back in my thoughts, knew what I was going to say and would finish sentences for me, and I felt I needed to establish myself as a person.'

Olivia's account of what was loving in her six year relationship with John was as follows:

Olivia: He made me feel the things I valued were valueless and I should be like him. He was very aware of the effect he was having and to everyone's amazement I was the one who eventually finished the relationship. That had a long-term effect on me. And I didn't feel I could cope with anything for a long time. I realized that although I thought the world of him, absolutely, I couldn't compromise, all the time.

When women became disaffected with particular relationships, the tendency did not seem to be for the men concerned to begin to meet them half-way in acceding to their emotional needs. Instead, only a joyless set of options for unilateral action seemed open, reflecting the degree to which the power relations were hierarchically set in men's favour. The women could end the relationship – as Sue was to do. They could accept the inevitability of such a situation fatalistically, as described by Zoë regarding the three or four long-term relationships she had been in with men. *Zoë*: 'Relationships deteriorate all the time in my experience. You kind of get taken for granted and the other one stops paying attention and being kind and considerate to you and that's almost kind of acceptable.'

Alternatively, women could retaliate. In the couple of cases where this involved violence to male partners on the part of the women concerned, even such apparently proactive behaviour was reactive. Without exonerating the women's behaviour, their accounts revealed the extent to which their actions had been driven by their partners' treatment of them. This was as opposed to women viewing their violence as part of their legitimate right to

dominate their partners, as in the male model of domestic violence eluci-
dated by the work of Dobash and Dobash (1980 and 1992).

> *Esther*: When the relationship finished, it was a complete shock to me,
> out of the blue. One day he did, then he couldn't bear to touch me . . .
> He didn't tell me he'd met somebody else, he just told me he wanted
> some space. Then three weeks later he told me . . . it evolved he wanted
> to screw this other woman without me around. One of us had to go
> away to sort things out so I went . . . then in the Autumn he went
> through the same spiel again, 'Oh God Esther, none of them are like
> you!' Then I discovered while he was saying all that, he was screwing
> this woman in Rotherham and having some sort of sexual relationship
> with this other woman that he'd left me for . . . I couldn't cope with the
> violence within me which had never surfaced before . . . I talked about
> it with friends, they said, 'It happens, you've had a lot of pent up feel-
> ings.' I screamed, walked round the house screaming, wanting to smash
> things, then eventually the thing I smashed was him. We were in my
> bedroom at the time, it must have been a terrible shock to him . . . I
> turned round and thumped him in the face and couldn't stop, it was
> awful.

> *Christine*: My husband felt that monogamous relationships concen-
> trated all the ills and you needed sexual relationships outside . . . and so
> we spent the first two years – he was still having a relationship with
> another woman – fighting, we fought verbally and by the time I got to
> the Centre I was hitting him. I was actually throwing him across the
> room . . .

Male partners' supportive behaviour

Women's accounts documented the negative effects of a variety of dominating tendencies in male partners' behaviour on their emotional wellbeing.
However, a minor theme in their accounts indicated that any critique of the
interaction of men's behaviour with women's emotional wellbeing needs to
take account of evidence of men's behaviour towards women being supportive as well as subordinating. Otherwise, there is the danger of crude stereo-
typing of all male behaviour as necessarily sexist, or as Hamblin (1983) has
argued, of dismissive treatment of women who perceive men's behaviour as
being at all-supportive, as suffering from false consciousness. In treading
this analytical path, however, care is needed to avoid falsely over-positive
readings of male behaviour as supportive, simply because it is not grossly
undermining. There is an element of this snare in Debbie's comments on her
second husband's behaviour. She praises him for not stunting her personal

development, which should be a basic human right – not an occasion for special gratitude.

> *Debbie*: My second husband: he's very good, lets me do what I want to do, he doesn't confine me, in fact he stretches me to do things. 'Yes she can do it, go on and do it.' He's very good like that.

With this caution in mind, several women nevertheless described how male partners had made a very positive contribution to their emotional wellbeing. Beatrice had been dogged by gynaecological problems and had recently undergone a mastectomy. She acknowledged niggling irritations in her marital relationship, but went on to describe her husband as 'fantastic, a most supportive partner' in the course of all she had had to face. Frances spoke of one of her four long-term heterosexual partners as providing 'an incredible amount of emotional support' as she tried to tackle the emotional vicissitudes which beset her. Mary described being in a relationship seemingly characterized by a good deal of emotional give and take.

> *Mary*: Whatever I say or do is OK. And if I'm actually pissed off with him I can say, 'Look I'm pissed off with you, I can't cope with this, I don't like what you're doing', and it gets sorted you know? I can be completely honest. I don't find it that easy but . . . sometimes . . . I know I'm going to say things that will hurt, but it's better to say it and get it sorted.

The phenomenon of the supportive male partner has been acknowledged in feminist writing but largely left untheorized except for hints that greater financial and legal independence for women may shift the balance in power relations between an individual woman and her male partner in her favour (Rowland 1993). There would seem to be further elements that require exploration in relation to the behaviour of both the man and the woman concerned than such analysis suggests. First, it is important not to assume that a supportive approach equals non-oppressive behaviour. Recent research has indicated, for example, that while men may endorse the idea of women's equality, men's engagement in routine childcare and domestic tasks is still minimal compared to that of their women partners (Witherspoon and Prior 1991). Despite this caveat, men's anti-sexist writings (e.g. Seidler 1991) have testified to the possibility of men as individuals being moved by contemporary feminism to try to act against the mainstream of sexist norms. However, men in our study were not identified by the women concerned as conspicuously anti-sexist. Therefore, the question is opened up of whether there is a hidden tradition of male resistance to gendered norms which is stronger than the discourse of the universality of macho attitudes suggests (McLeod 1982: Ch. 3; Morgan 1992: Ch. 1).

Improvements in a woman's individual material circumstances may neutralize the gendered power balance between her and her male partner, helping to induce a more supportive approach. This seemed to have occurred in Mary's case: she related that prior to her current relationship she had adopted a subordinate role in heterosexual relationships. *Mary*: 'I think then I was very caring . . . so I was filling that role where if they wanted anything I would do it . . . it was OK, it was what I was there to do . . . but now I wasn't locked in that sort of role any more.' Between her previous heterosexual relationship and her current more equitable one, she had been on her own for five years. She had gained financial independence and did not want to change that. However, the chance of a woman being able to gain such a great degree of individual material independence is related to other dimensions of social inequality, such as her class position (Ramazanoglou 1989: Ch. 5).

Women's dominating behaviour

Women's accounts also suggested that they could behave in a dominating way in heterosexual relationships. However, some instances of such behaviour could be seen as being retaliatory, as in Esther and Christine's case, with the course of the relationship still basically set on their male partners' terms. Although evidence from women's partners was not available as a preliminary to analysis, there was also evidence of dominating behaviour on women's part which disregarded partner's interests, without apparent provocation.

> *Irene*: I don't think I was very nice to him most of the time. Because I was depressed for quite a number of periods in that relationship, I have a feeling I played an awful lot of games with him, to be putting him into no-win situations, and sort of using him as my punchbag really . . . He took it [surprise]. He seemed to feel there must be an end to it all, sometime, and he just wanted to wait for it all to end so I could go back to being what I was when I first met him. So he seemed prepared to take an awful lot.

Acknowledging that women can behave in a dominating way opens up the possibility of greater understanding of the nature and effects of such behaviour. Otherwise, the discovery that such behaviour exists can simply be used to trivialize men's dominating behaviour on the grounds that women also engage in this (Dobash and Dobash 1992: Ch. 8). Without condoning Irene's behaviour, the indications are that ironically the disablist and ageist treatment she had as a child may have contributed to her persistent feelings of unhappiness that fed into how she behaved. At the same time, the tone of these comments – her surprise that her partner 'took it' – are reflective of her continuing incredulity that anyone could accept her, which also seemed to emanate from her experience in childhood (see Chapter 2). Meanwhile, there is a hint in her account that her partner was into the politics of the 'waiting game'.

Finally, there was some evidence of women setting the terms in heterosexual relationships – as in an initiative on Gillian's part – where it did not seem appropriate to read the behaviour as dominating, so much as assertive: the woman concerned ensuring that her interests were also met. Gillian's male partner Grant had left her and their child precipitately and with no explanation. However, by the time he had returned, wanting to restart the relationship, Gillian had changed the balance of power through her actions.

> *Gillian*: I started looking for jobs, got one, put her [her daughter] in the nursery and just carried on from there. I said 'Well, Grant, you sorted out your life, now I've sorted out mine.' When he did want to come back, my love had just gone, because I was too wrapped up in thinking about looking for a better house, got this place and things I'd like to get and the only way I could get the things was to work. And by working I didn't have time to think about him. And it just died out of my life.

A slight improvement in Gillian's class position *vis-à-vis* her male partner through her entering employment can be seen as germane to this change in the balance of power.

The further impact of other dimensions to social inequality

Other dimensions to social inequality than gender may have been implicated in apparent exceptions to the gendered rule in heterosexual relationships. They also compounded the gendered nature of such relationships as well as having an impact in their own right. These tendencies are illustrated in Winifred's and Annie's accounts. In Winifred's case the gendered assumption and practice that she would be the prime carer (Graham 1993) has already been referred to. However, the disablist dearth of social provision to underwrite the independence of people with disabilities, legitimated by the ideology that caring is appropriately carried out 'in the family' with the minimum of state funded support (Oliver 1990), can be seen as inextricably interwoven with this. The effects on Winifred's emotional wellbeing were dire:

> Because of the absolute time a handicapped child takes, you don't go out because it's very rarely you can get a baby sitter who's got the sense to know what to do . . . I spent a lot of my time while Kim was at home sleeping to catch up, every afternoon because at night I'd have to get up about every half hour. You imagine being conditioned to never sleeping . . . I lost so much of my life.

Annie, in her mid-fifties, had recently experienced a host of troubles in her life, relating to her own health and that of her daughter and her work. In addition, as a result of constant medication for high blood pressure, her husband had become impotent. Annie had greatly valued their sexual relationship and wanted advice on how best to continue it in some form. However, she had found it impossible to gain such advice informally or formally because of ageist assumptions desexualizing older people (Kitzinger 1985: Ch. 7) and felt a great sense of loss:

> *Annie*: I feel that an ideal relationship could go on indefinitely, I don't see why it should stop because of age or anything else, because you feel the same inside. The fact that sexual relationships are not talked about for older people – it doesn't mean they don't continue. It's just that people don't talk about it.

Lesbian relationships

A shift in focus

Women's accounts illustrated how it is also essential to give an account of lesbian experience and heterosexism as interacting with gender when analysing the significant factors contributing to women's emotional wellbeing. From women's experience, the pre-eminence of heterosexual relationships clearly rested not only on the gendered nature of social relations but their heterosexist nature as well. In turn, the marginalization of lesbian relations reflected the effects of both sexism and heterosexism at work.

Wilkinson and Kitzinger have argued that part of the ideological process underpinning heterosexism is that lesbianism is interrogated from a heterosexist standpoint. It has to explain itself from a heterosexist norm, for example, as 'alternative lifestyle' at best, 'pathological perversion' at worst (1993: 1). They advocate a reversal of this process so that heterosexuality is interrogated in the interests of legitimating lesbianism (1993: 1–26). Several women in our sample had had or currently were in lesbian relationships. Their experience already embodied the shift in focus that Wilkinson and Kitzinger argue for – to the extent that lesbian relationships were the yardstick by which they judged other relationships. *Christine*: 'The most loving relationships I've had in the past have been with women.' *Ruth*: 'A relationship with another woman is like being a mother and a baby all at once, it's marvellous, it really is nice.' In describing their engagement in lesbian relations, other women brought out how for them this had fundamentally transformed their personality – enabling them to express themselves as never before. *Tina*: 'I found it affected everything I did and how I saw the world. It completely changed my outlook on the world.'

> *Jan*: A major breakthrough in relationships came when I first got involved with a woman when I was 25 – this was someone I'd been very

emotionally close to and talked to a lot about very personal things . . . I haven't ever treated men I've been involved with as friends . . . They were people I slept with, but they weren't people I felt any closeness with.

Heterosexism undermining emotional wellbeing

While women experienced lesbian relationships as so intrinsically rewarding, the heterosexist nature of social relations had undermined or continued to undermine their emotional wellbeing. For example, although Ruth was to gain such happiness in lesbian relations, the existing taboo on lesbianism had made it difficult to find out in practice about its existence and how to meet other lesbian women.

Ruth: I always felt I wanted a special friend and it's in the past six or seven years I realized I wanted a close friendship, and I wasn't sure what sort of friendship I wanted but there was a need to put my arms around and touch a woman and of course it's very difficult.

Tina described breaking through a similar process of social and interpersonal taboo:

I didn't realise it till I thought about it, why I wasn't bothered about going out with men . . . But it never occurred to me that because I couldn't have men I could have women . . . It was like a big thing. I didn't know a lot about the lesbian scene, it's ridiculous all this literature there is, I wasn't even aware . . . you see my life revolved around my job and I wasn't mixing in social circles broadly enough to be aware that there were women who appreciated other women's friendships.

Tina's experience also illustrated how heterosexism undermines non-sexual close relationships as well. She had come out to her family as gay, but the stigma attached to lesbian and gay identity had led to her estrangement from them despite the fact that she clearly yearned for their support.

Tina: They (my family) know I'm gay. I suppose I should discuss it with them a lot . . . but it seems very much I've got different influences from them. It's right for me to be away from them, because I am very different now . . . I fear being rejected in some way or being made to feel inadequate or strange or whatever.

In other women's experience the stigma attached to lesbianism was so all-pervasive, that it had resulted in the tension of them denying their lesbian sexual identity to themselves and pathologizing it, although they had found it to be their truest form of self-expression. *Nina*: 'It's quite difficult to accept, other than knowing that they [lesbian partners] are there and I love them and need it and want it. I don't think I accepted that about myself until I went to the Therapy Centre.' *Esther*: 'I worry about what people think, you are worried about what people think if you're normal. I don't think of myself as being gay, I just think I love Chris, which is different isn't it? A cop out . . .'.

Nearly all the women who nominated lesbian relationships as the most important or among the most important in their adult lives had also had heterosexual relationships. In several instances (Christine, Irene, Nina, Ruth and Esther), they described lesbian relationships as having been more satisfying than the heterosexual relationships around which they had organized their public life. For example, Esther commented on her response to a man who had wanted to marry her.

> *Esther*: I didn't say to him, 'I'm not interested in you because I'm having this really good time with X' [her lesbian partner], and that wasn't actually what I was thinking, because what he was offering was very tempting: a normal respectable comfortable future. But I didn't really see that as a reality.

The way in which the women shrank back from giving public recognition to their lesbian relationships could be seen as both a response to and as contributing to the vicious circle whereby lesbian relations are marginalized and stigmatized as a deviant world apart, despite their central importance to the women immediately involved.

Sites of caring and dominating behaviour

Women also referred to lesbian relationships as characterized by elements of very caring behaviour. This contrasted with the tendency towards male–female hierarchies of need in heterosexual relationships. *Tina*: 'I think they [lesbian relationships] are far more sensitive to needs, women tend to be far more supportive to each other, interested, I don't know.' This tendency was also reflected in women's statements about their own behaviour: *Esther*, on her first lesbian partner: 'I was very worried about using her to find out about my sexuality. Which has worried me. I talked this over with her. She was willing to take the risk . . . we had really nice times together.'

Notwithstanding these positive attributes, women's comments also revealed that lesbian relationships were sites of dominating behaviour. Tina, ruminating on her own participation in the lesbian scene, commented on how women could treat other women as sex objects and subjects for domination:

> *Tina*: There's a lot of objectifying women, men do it, but women do it a lot too, a meat market a bit, sometimes, which shocked me . . . the butch and femme types. You can find that, but there's also many other 'different' kinds of relationships. Some stay together – adult and equal

relationships, other are parent/child power struggles. But I think there are people who like to play the dominant role.

Although she was currently in a lesbian relationship which she felt had produced great happiness and a flowering of her personality, Nina had previously experienced intensely dominating behaviour from a lesbian partner. The woman concerned could also not accept that their relationship had ended. Besides harassing Nina by persistently waylaying her and subjecting her to verbal abuse, she had smashed windows in her house. *Nina's* comments indicated the state of subjection she had been driven to, 'I tried to convince myself that I had rights, that I was a person.'

There has been growing recognition of the existence of dominating behaviour in lesbian relationships, focusing on such phenomena as lesbian and sado-masochistic sexual behaviour (Ardill and O'Sullivan 1986) and women's physical abuse of other women (Lobel 1986). The origins of such behaviour remains unclear and I cannot comment from a position within lesbian relationships. However, Kelly has argued that ironically such behaviour may represent an extension of the role model of male dominance – employing violence to assert control:

> What I am suggesting here is that in rejecting traditional femininity, lesbians may borrow from or identify with aspects of heterosexual and/or gay masculinity in order to construct a sense of self; and that these identifications might in some way explain a lesbian's choice to use physical force against her lover.
>
> (Kelly 1991: 19)

In arguing this point, Kelly conceptualizes lesbian women's behaviour as though it is 'model driven', i.e. as though the model of behaviour itself comes to set the course of their future actions. This line of argument may be correct, but it begs certain questions. While the male role incorporates violence to women as one of its hallmarks, it is not without exception violent, therefore in adopting it there is no absolute necessity to be violent. Without overwhelming proof to the contrary, it is also possible to question whether women's desire to behave in a violent or dominating way towards other women may precede their choice of role or parts of that role. Moreover, it may be that the interplay of different aspects of social inequality is present in another way. A point that Kelly also raises in passing is that violence between lesbian women may be a reflection of social divisions between them (Kelly 1991: 19). However, systematic evidence on this issue does not seem to be available.

The significance of women's childhood experience and children's comparative powerlessness

The legacy of childhood experience

A substantial number of the women in our sample had testified to their childhood experience as significantly undermining their self-esteem and thereby their capacity to pursue their own interests through subsequent relationships. However, women's accounts of the interaction between this dimension to their experience and initiatives by other parties to relationships in adulthood indicated that it did not determine their emotional wellbeing in an over-riding way. Childhood experience played its part, but so did other people's behaviour, the influence of wider social conditions and the existing or developing capacity for self-expression and assertiveness of the women themselves.

Relatively unproblematic childhood relationships did not necessarily result in positive experiences of adult relationships in adulthood. For instance, Esther described affectionate responsive relations with parents, leaving no legacy of damaged self-esteem, but had been driven to doubting her own sanity as a result of dismissive treatment from a male partner. Moreover, despite constant probing in the course of counselling, she was adamant that the roots of her adult tribulations did not lie in childhood experiences.

Where women described childhood experience as leaving them inclined to subordinate the importance of their own emotional wellbeing in subsequent relationships, this did not guarantee exploitation by others. Debbie, spoke of how friends in adulthood had had a positive effect on the precarious nature of her feelings of selfworth. *Debbie*: 'They've stabilized me a lot, it's difficult to say . . . if I'd been without them . . . they mean an awful lot to me . . . it would be an unbearable thought.' Jan described feelings of emotional closeness for the first time in a lesbian relationship when she was 25, as breaching the consistent loneliness of a sense of emotional distance from others acquired during childhood. Moreover, women also described how, despite the damage previously incurred to their self-esteem, in the comparatively egalitarian conditions of certain heterosexual and lesbian relationships and friendships, their capacity for self-expression and assertiveness had flowered. As *Olivia*, referring to her friendship, put it:

> I think it's probably the most supportive relationship I've ever had . . . I can be myself with Gill. Sometimes I've been in an incredibly dreadful state, but I can be myself, that's the important thing.

Where women's emotional vulnerability acquired in childhood was faced with dominating behaviour from the other party in a relationship, there was some evidence that the negative effects of the dominating behaviour could be amplified, exacerbating the unhappiness that was caused. It was as though the woman was going into hostile territory already wounded. This was a feature of heterosexual relationships but not unique to them. Thus Winifred's preoccupation with putting others' needs first, instilled in childhood, was met in marriage by a husband who was only too happy to let her do so – resulting in a lifetime literally lived for others which had left her chronically depressed.

Gillian described how, despite her childhood experience of sexual abuse and the resultant feeling of being scared to love, she had trusted, confided in and loved Grant. *Gillian*: 'He know's me. He know's what I've been through, what colours I like . . . I did love him I really did.' He then left her abruptly and for no given reason. At the time she had shown considerable fortitude. *Gillian*: 'I thought I can't stay like this for the rest of my life, shut in the house, there's my little girl, can't spend the rest of my life on the social . . . go out and get a job.' She had set the terms when Grant had tried to come back (see p. 64). Her love for Grant had also now died. However, the experience had also clearly shaken Gillian's confidence profoundly. She described how Grant had been the only person she had let into her 'secret life':

> *Gillian*: I don't want to tell anybody else because he buggered off and left me. I don't want anybody else to do that. And I just don't want to be alone anymore. So rather than get involved with somebody who'll leave me, I don't get involved at all. That's the effect, it scares me at times.

Nina described how a relationship in which the other woman had resorted to psychological and physical harassment to assert control had fomented Nina's persistent lack of self-confidence from childhood. The result had been to leave Nina feeling almost overwhelmed to the point of losing her self-identity.

Relationships with parents in adulthood

In addition to the role that parent–child relationships played through the legacy of childhood experience, relationships with parents themselves in adulthood emerged as having a significant influence. In doing so they seemed to be characterized by earlier features of the exercise of parental power spanning the spectrum of the benign to the authoritarian. Parents were still turned to as an important source of material and emotional support (Willmott 1987). *Esther* commented on the continuing benefits of her relationship with her parents. They did things

> like having the children – so I could go away without [them], when I was having an operation – just being there . . . when this young bloke

appeared, I thought they'd never speak to me again, but in fact they were very supportive and understanding.

In this context, the death of a parent could represent an acute loss of someone who was a profound source of and focus of love. Louise, who cried in the interview as she thought of her father who had died four years previously, described a continuing process of emotional and material support. *Louise*: 'Dad was always around when there were jobs to be done, helping out, financially, with transport, with the children.'

In some instances adulthood evened up the balance of power in parent–child relationships that had been very injurious, but the behaviour of the woman concerned was still marked by earlier events – as in Gillian's wary approach to her abusing stepfather:

Gillian: I do it for my mum's sake – I go to my mums with a plastic face while he's there, a plastic smile, plastic talk, I don't want to be there – but I want to see my mum and my brothers and I don't want him to stop me from seeing them so he's there but he isn't.

The most extreme example of a parent's continuing hold over the conduct of a child in a relationship in adulthood was provided by Winifred's experience. Objectively, Winifred's mother, although fit, was very dependent on Winifred's discretion as to how much she helped her, Winifred being more mobile and having more financial resources. Prior to contact with the Centre this was not how Winifred had felt however. Winifred's situation can be seen as mediated by the gendered expectation that younger women relatives will assume the prime responsibility of caring for older single parents (Pitkeathly, 1989). However, she had still experienced the same sense of utter account-ability for her mother's wellbeing – however much she resented its demands – as she had reported feeling in childhood. Discussing the effect of contact with the Therapy Centre on her attitude, *Winifred* commented, 'I was in a position of not being able to say no to Mother – she [the counsellor] helped me to cope with my mother a bit and to know it isn't my complete responsibility.'

Women's relationships with their own children

Turning to women's experience as adults of relationships with their own children confirmed the significance of the gendered nature of these relation-ships for women's emotional wellbeing. The ten women who had children, without exception, described relations with them as important in terms of their parental responsibility. For example, *Katherine*, referring to her daughter as a key person in her life: 'I love her, feel responsible for her and protect her.' *Gillian*: 'There's my little girl, I need to fend for her.' Embedded in several of their accounts was the delineation of maternal responsibility as conceived and practised more generally, with prime responsibility for caring falling on women as mothers, whose self-sacrifice was an integral and appropriate part of motherhood (Graham 1993). The balance between satisfaction and self-sacrifice women described in discharging such a role varied – Louise hinted at some regrets.

Louise: And of course the children, Diane and Jim, are extremely important. Although I've spent a semi-professional life, they've always come first, probably because of that I've missed one or two chances.

In Winifred's case the demands of bringing up a child with profound learning difficulties had reduced her to a state of chronic physical and emotional exhaustion.

Winifred: I don't know whether if I'd known what I was in for I'd have even started. My conscience is absolutely clear, I've done my level best . . . People say you should be very proud of this, and in a way I am, but I did it for my child Kim, I didn't get anything out of this . . . It's part of my frustration . . . So that's been hell on earth and probably affected my life more than anything really . . .

However, the women's accounts also testified to the influence of the phenomenon of children's comparative powerlessness as being in play. For example, a couple of the women discussed how as a central feature of their interaction with their children, they had tried to loosen up the stereotypical parent–child roles which they had experienced in childhood. Their aim was that their children's emotional welfare and their own as parents would benefit from what they saw as a more egalitarian approach. Ironically, through their descriptions they revealed the hierarchical assumption on which they were operating – that the power differential was theirs to employ to influence their children.

Mary: With my children – especially my son – I'm not prepared to get into that role with him he's got to become independent. And my daughter – I don't want them to feel about me the way I felt about my mother, it's a fine balance and I'm still trying to find that. The caring role and the nurturing parent, and sort of more independent.

Katherine: I parented her totally different to my parents . . . just actually the opposite. I was determined, I suppose, at a very early stage to avoid what went wrong with me and I was determined it wasn't going to happen to her . . . so she is totally different to how I am, as a result.

Most significantly for women's emotional wellbeing in adulthood, the phenomenon of children's comparative powerlessness seemed to affect their relationships with their own children in another way. Of the ten women with children, none of the six who did cite their relationships with them as among the most important in their adult life, did so on the basis of describing the emotional relationship which their children offered as being equal to that offered by adults. This may simply have reflected the influence of ideological assumptions among adults that children are not their equals emotionally (Miller 1988; 1989). Such a situation may also have reflected the low expectations with which the women's own treatment in childhood had left them. At best they had been treated benignly, though not as on a par with their parents. At worst what they could offer adults emotionally in a relationship had been grossly undervalued. However, it meant that even on the rare occasions when women did acknowledge that what affection their children offered approached what adults could offer, they did not identify such an offering as characteristic of children. Instead they immediately translated it into an adult-like gesture. *Esther*, speaking of her daughter: 'She's almost an adult now, she's 18 . . . the last relationship was the one that caused my downfall, why I had to go to therapy, she was just fantastic, it was like having another woman in the house, all of a sudden she grew up.'

> *Katherine*: Cheryl [her daughter] gives me a feeling of satisfaction, she loves me and cares about me . . . I won't let her be responsible for me, sometimes I feel she wants to be – it's more adult to adult now rather than parent to child.

From what we know of what children do offer from the women's own accounts of when they were younger, this lack of recognition would seem to result in a poignant loss for women of an important source of enriching affection.

Relationships with women friends

Introduction

Women's comments suggested that the remaining type of relationship which they identified as among the most important to them, friendship with other women, was the most consistent source of emotional validation. It compared well with the main tendencies of heterosexual relationships, with parent–child relationships, women's adult experience of parent–child relationships and, in some instances, lesbian relationships. The only exceptions to women friends being identified as important were provided by Beatrice, who identified family relationships as her primary source of emotional support, and by some other cases discussed subsequently, where other parties were identified as providing sources of friendship rated as important.

Questions of definition

Rubin, in one of the few systematic surveys of women's and men's friendships, has indicated that what is defined as friendship covers myriad experiences in terms of differing forms and degrees of formality, status, intimacy, durability and reciprocity. Moreover, that 'friendship' or having friends may also have an idealized or symbolic value as a form of personal assurance or public affirmation that our wellbeing has adequate protection (Rubin 1985: Ch. 1). Her findings also argue against assuming that one party's valuation of a friendship should be assumed to represent its nature for both those involved. Where her original interviews led her to have some doubts about the reciprocity of the relationships involved in friendship, she asked to be referred on to all the people who had been identified as close friends or best friends. When contacting these people she found 64 per cent made no mention on their list of friends of the person she originally interviewed (Rubin 1985: 6). This is an important caution to bear in mind in terms of our findings where we only interviewed one party.

Despite the inherent difficulties in pin-pointing the true nature of relationships defined as friendships, as reflected in Rubin's study, her findings also indicate that amongst accounts of friendships a group of relationships emerge which seem to merit the title of 'best friends'. This signifies 'a level of attachment, of intimacy, of commitment, of sharing that transcends all other friendships' (Rubin 1985: 178). While the women we interviewed indicated that they saw positive benefits accruing generally from their friendships with other women, the friendships they referred to as among the most important relationships in their lives seemed to equate with this typification of 'best friends'.

These friendships took no set form. In several cases women referred to such friendships as consisting of one-to-one contacts with other women they were unrelated to but saw frequently. However, for example, Nina referred to women friends with whom she rarely had contact as nevertheless being very important to her emotional wellbeing. *Nina*: 'I might not see them often, but just knowing they are there.' Friendships could also mutate into other forms of relationships as in *Jan*'s case – 'She was actually a friend who I gradually fell in love with . . . this was someone I'd been very emotionally close to and talked to a lot about very personal things.' In two or three cases such as Katherine's, a relationship with a sister seemed to fulfil a very similar role to that of best friend. *Katherine*: 'She's the one I share a lot with and I'm not used to sharing, I'm very selective . . . She's the one I trust the most and I feel whatever I do in terms of telling my sister, or her finding out, it doesn't affect how she feels about me, it's OK.' O'Connor's review of studies of women's friendships (1992: Ch. 6) indicates that while women did not necessarily identify sisters as best friends, in several surveys they featured prominently as occupying this role. Moreover, her own work also found that such closeness was much more likely to characterize close sister–sister, than mother–daughter relationships.

In a few instances women identified men as best friends. *Esther*: 'and I do feel loved by three men friends whom I love deeply . . . who have been very supportive to me, and I've gone and cried on their shoulder at two in the morning and they haven't turned me away.' Swain (1992) has commented that the social support of heterosexual coupling and same sex friendships means that such cross-sex friendships can be considered a somewhat subversive activity. Certainly women who referred to having male friends registered this as containing an element of the unusual, as in Esther's comments here. In the minority of cases where women had spoken positively of heterosexual relationships, they had also indicated that these had qualities akin to their relationships with women friends, such as acceptance and endorsement of their individual identity and worth rather than its subordination, with positive consequences for their self-esteem. With this in mind, perhaps friendships should be defined even more fluidly.

On the other hand, lesbian feminist interest in the issue of lesbian identity has raised the issue of whether women can authentically relate to each other if they are 'male identified', that is obtaining status through attachment to and association with men (Wilkinson and Kitzinger 1993). If this perspective is adhered to, then many of the friendships women identified as such in our sample would be regarded as being of suspect value for their emotional wellbeing and not worthy of the term.

Positive benefits

Women described their friendships with other women as providing a high degree of acceptance, which in turn made a high degree of self-expression possible. Women characterized them as being based on a greater degree of give and take than heterosexual relationships and also as comparatively dependable. They saw them as having very positive effects on their emotional wellbeing. On her friendship with a fellow woman teacher at school:

Olivia: We have a very close and important relationship because I can talk to her about almost anything, and it's mutual . . . We don't go out socially, her social circle is completely different to mine, but we're still friends. Just generally I know I can rely on her if I need moral support and that's very important.

Debbie, on one particular friend: 'Her husband left her for a short time and I've been through that. You can start talking about anything' and on her women friends in general, 'I hope I've always been as supportive as they've been to me . . .' *Sue*: 'I've had one or two close friends, girlfriends – who I've always been able to talk to and they've provided stability in my life.'

> *Zoë*: As far as receiving love, I'd say I get that more from my relationships with female friends than I do from my male friends, because they tend to be nice to you, they don't take it out on you. You're not there as their emotional sounding board.

The picture of the positive benefits for women's emotional health of a confiding relationship emerging from the women's accounts here, echoes the findings of Brown, Andrews, Harris, et al. (1986), that such support from 'a very close tie' was associated with a low risk of depression among married women. It also reflects O'Connor's findings – that women with a confidante were less likely to have an affective disorder (O'Connor 1992: 84). It is tempting to conclude that what seems to be the relatively egalitarian nature of the relationship between women and their women friends provides them with just the sort of emotional benefits they require and therefore should be regarded as unproblematic. However, without denying the benefits that women describe, the situation is more complex than that.

Problematic aspects to women's friendships

Raymond has criticized the mutually confiding relationship informing women's friendships on several grounds. First, investing their energies in such friendships tends to deflect women from asserting themselves in public life and the wider world of work. Second, women feel it incumbent on them to make their feelings manifest, as opposed to refining their own thoughts as an aid to originality. 'Relationism, or the relationship centredness of women, is an obstacle to female friendship because it draws women's energy away from herself, her original friend, always to others' (Raymond 1986: 161). Third, the *raison d'être* of these friendships tends to be the constant discussion and re-examination of relationships focusing on another person. In this way the friendships serve to confirm 'the relationship-centredness of many women, heterosexual or lesbian [which] makes others the centre of a woman's life' (Raymond 1986: 161).

Our findings tend to contradict Raymond's arguments in several ways. None of the women suggested that the only topic of conversation within their friendships was other relationships. Our study was not designed to establish whether or not the women concerned would have pursued careers or their careers more ambitiously without their friendships with other women. What it is possible to say is that all the women who identified such relationships as important did waged work, and their comments in one or two instances indicated that the support of women friends was crucial to sustaining them in this. Esther on a particular woman friend:

Esther: When she went to Africa, I spent a couple of years at a total loss. I didn't have another woman friend that I could talk to, so all my worries and problems – it was my probationary year as a teacher – were on this bloke I was living with. It was a bad time, and we used to have long discussions. 'Oh God, it's not my fault, it's Mary she shouldn't have gone to Africa, I've got nobody else except you.'

In some instances women also specifically commented on how friendships with other women had opened up their understanding of the world. *Annie* described how a friendship with a woman which had arisen out of a reciprocal childcare arrangement developed her own understanding of childrearing: 'in that my mother's rather rigid view of it was not hers . . . it was a way of moving forward which I wouldn't have otherwise had.' Winifred also commented on how after her restrictive upbringing, a friend's mother had become a friend and moral lodestar, who opened her eyes after her restrictive upbringing to the wider range of guilt-free conduct women could engage in.

While not endorsing Raymond's arguments, our findings indicated that in certain respects women's friendships with other women were problematic. The experience of women in our study – that their most sustaining relationship tended to be with women friends and not with their own male partner, was in keeping with Hite's survey (1987) where the majority of women respondents with male partners had found the same. However, given the pre-eminent position of heterosexual relationships in society, this suggests that women's friendships may be fulfilling a compensatory role – maintaining heterosexual relationships by catering for emotional needs they fail to provide. In this way women's friendships may actually be functioning in the longer term to perpetuate the dominance of a form of relationship inimical to women's wellbeing. Some further empirical support for this comes from Oliker's study of married women's friendships with other women. The majority of married women in her study commented that such friendships had buttressed their marital relationship by providing a safety valve for negative feelings, as well as providing affection which had been lacking in their marriages (1989).

If the role of difference between women in relation to the basis for friendship is also not explored, then there is a danger of falling into the trap of assuming that it is simply a common sisterhood which fuels women's friendship. As a result, differences that may exclude women from each other's friendship may be overlooked. Women's friendships – as in regard to our sample – could be examples of great social homogeneity in terms of the women concerned, but thereby could represent the exclusion of the possibility of friendships with women who did not occupy a position of social equivalence. An example of this process in operation is offered by Cohen's work on women's networks on a suburban middle-class estate. Cohen (1978) found that women's friendship networks served to minimize internal differences between the women involved, but accentuated differences between them and other women from other social classes outside the estate.

If women's friendships tend to reinforce existing social divisions between women, then our study suggests that the interaction of elements of equality and inequality in power relations at a particular point in time, which may be germane to a friendship forming, is subtle and complex. This is illustrated in Olivia's description of how her close friendship came about. It would be difficult to account for the state of loneliness and desperation in which Olivia turned to her future friend, without reference to the effects on Olivia of the hierarchical relationships she had experienced in childhood, implicated for her in the onset of bulimia. It would also be difficult to account for both Olivia and her future friend being in the same occupation, without some reference to their respective social backgrounds. It is difficult to account for her future friend's stigmatized position within the staff group and the levelling-up effect that Olivia confiding in her had, without knowledge of the way in which the effects of existing social divisions had coalesced in her friend's experience and self-image.

> *Olivia*: Well, we teach in the same school, and for six years I didn't really know her, but she was always very much a loner as regards staff room type relationships, very much mocked – not quite the word [pause] – just talked about behind her back. There was one particular occasion at school, I was incredibly depressed, and just had got to talk to someone . . . good cry, apologized for unloading my troubles on her and she was so pleased I was able to talk to her, she kind of set up the beginnings of a friendship. And when I left the school she came for tea and it developed from there really. We have a very close and important relationship because I can talk to her about anything, and its mutual. We're not at all alike, we're like chalk and cheese. We don't go out socially, her social circle is completely different to mine, but we're still friends.

If participation in friendships between women embodies some idea of equivalence of investment on the part of both parties, then this may be problematic if a disparity develops between the demands that each party needs to make. Such a disparity could arise if the emotional difficulties individuals are facing are so engulfing that they legitimately require undivided attention. This danger is reflected in *Christine*'s comment: 'Friends are fine but I think there comes a point when friends get fed up at being used as sounding boards, they've got their own needs to be met themselves.'

O'Connor (1992) has also stressed the limitations of defining friendships as just being about 'feelings', arguing instead that they are maintained by work – on such things as arranging contact, investment of energy and time.

Therefore, if one party is unable to sustain her input of these things as a result of being in a debilitated emotional state, or because of other demands on her time, or shortage of resources, then her hold on friendships with other women may be very tenuous, or dissolve. Winifred's comparative isolation from women friends illustrated this problem. In doing so, it reflected the pattern of informal carers finding it extremely difficult to get a break from their responsibilities in order to have any social life of their own (Spackman 1991: 10).

> *Winifred*: Since I've had Kim [her child with learning difficulties] I've been rather lonely, I haven't had women friends, I haven't really got many women friends now, I don't really go out and do much, I've only just started to go out and do things now.

Despite their evident blessings, the female friendships enjoyed by women in our sample cannot therefore simply be treated as a panacea for women's emotional wellbeing. Indications of their conservative and exclusive tendencies together with their negotiated status suggest that they should also be considered as having problematic aspects.

Conclusion: Limitations to analysing women's emotional wellbeing, in terms of subordination through gender

The experience across childhood and adulthood of women in our sample shows that it is essential to take account of the gendered nature of women's emotional wellbeing. However, this is also constantly mediating and being mediated by the effects of other dimensions to inequality such as heterosexism and children's comparative powerlessness. Their experience also suggests that in childhood and adulthood, women's psychology cannot be characterized by self-denying passivity, but instead that they retain a capacity for self-expression and assertiveness, although this may be overlaid or undermined by the impact of hierarchical social relations. There were also indications of women having a capacity for dominating behaviour.

The experience of women in the sample also suggests that the closer women come to enjoying a situation of comparative equality in any relationship, the more their emotional wellbeing flowers. This is as a result of their need for affection being more likely to be met, their care and affection for other people being more likely to be valued, and they themselves being more likely to value the care and affection others offer. Women's 'best friendships' emerge as the most likely site where these conditions obtain. However, even such relationships seem questionable – with a tendency to reinforce existing hierarchies and prone to dissolution by them.

four

A big struggle to change: counsellors' experience of feminist therapy

Introduction

In this chapter and the next, feminist therapy is analysed as a relationship in the context of other relationships in women's lives. It is also analysed in the context of the evidence so far on the nature of women's emotional resources and needs and the social conditions implicated in them.

Here, the views and experience of the counsellors and coordinator of a specific feminist therapy centre are examined to illuminate the approach of practitioners more generally. This is essential as a preliminary to analysing the significance of feminist therapy for women participants. It is also important in its own right: both to provide a fair assessment of what counsellors are aiming to do, and to take account of how their work affects their own emotional wellbeing.

The theories the counsellors referred to and their account of their activities are analysed to determine how egalitarian their approach seems to be. First, the extent to which their theoretical framework for practice took account of the need to tackle profound social inequalities is reviewed. Second, the degree to which they defined women as co-workers in feminist therapy as opposed to subordinates is discussed. Finally, the Centre's organization as a model of equity, is analysed.

Theoretical frames of reference

The structure and content of the counsellors' theoretical framework had much in common with that in practitioners' accounts generally (Ernst and Maguire 1987; Walker 1990). It did not take the form of a single theory with internal coherence. Instead it was an amalgam of several distinctive perspectives found on a widespread basis in feminist therapy. These were:

- a feminist perspective;
- an awareness of social divisions other than gender;
- a psychotherapeutic approach;
- a commitment to the ideals and forms of intervention identified as present in counselling.

An examination of the theoretical frames of reference in this Centre is therefore an examination of a microcosm of some of the main theoretical tendencies in feminist therapy at large.

Each of the main perspectives the counsellors adopted had its own strengths and weaknesses in taking account of the need to tackle profound social inequalities. In some respects diverse theories complemented each other. But allegiance to any one could also occlude continuing consciousness of the insights of another. This did not mean that the counsellors were theoretical dilettantes. Rather, that they were at a particular stage in the evolution of their theory making. A variety of different factors also influenced their theoretical framework. Personal commitment to certain ideals, experience in certain lines of analysis, some deeply entrenched working practices and the powerful impact of clients' experience formed the kaleidoscopic way in which various theoretical perspectives were 'held'.

Each of the main perspectives informing the counsellors' work and the extent to which it took account of the need to tackle profound social inequalities is now discussed in turn.

Tackling profound social inequalities – a feminist perspective

The counsellors' and coordinator's commitment

The counsellors' commitment to a feminist perspective seemed profound in that it was deeply rooted in their personal experience. In keeping with a pattern common in feminist activism (Dominelli and McLeod 1989: Ch. 2), they had all become involved in the Centre as a result of their growing awareness of what they perceived to be feminist ideals, together with their allegiance to them, leading to their engagement in collective action. This process was exemplified in the lives of all the counsellors but epitomized in Miriam's and Fran's accounts.

Miriam: I was becoming active in the women's liberation movement as a result of a violent incident directed against me . . . I decided [that] there was in X – unlike [what] the articles I read in magazines, said there was in London – no women's group which was particularly looking at models

of women's psychology which took account of the insights of feminism...
I understood them in a very crude way, but I was quite angry about what
I discovered to be passing as knowledge about women's emotional
life . . . I got together with a group of women who started a women's
therapy group . . . I put out a publicity sheet to gather women together
and as a result ten women met, it must have been about 1974. That
group ran and I was a member of it until about 1982.

Fran: I was finding in feminist literature, actually written down what I'd
already known on some level, like an incredible confirmation process
and affirmation . . . developing those ideas in my professional work . . .
my personal life at home, changing an awful lot there.

On then being invited to join in the group that led to the Centre being set up,
Fran said, 'It was like being in a place where you really wanted to be.'

Bridget, the coordinator's, personal commitment seemed just as deep as
that of the counsellors, but it was to women's interests and socialist ideas as
opposed to an explicitly feminist perspective.

Bridget: I think the work of the Centre is about empowering women –
giving them a sense of value in themselves. But I think that women have
that in common with a lot of men . . . I felt it would be good to be
working with women.

In this way also, the pattern of commitment amongst the workers at the
Centre as members of a feminist collective was similar to that reported in
feminist literature more generally, i.e. a broad spectrum of commitment
involving differences in degree and kind (Donnelly 1986).

The sexist nature of social relations

The counsellors' account of feminist therapy was imbued with concern about
sexist social relations. *Miriam*: 'If I were going to make just two statements I
would say feminist therapy understands women's psychology in the context
of patriarchy and misogyny and would identify power as a key issue.' The
counsellors identified the gendered nature of childhood relationships as
having important consequences for women's emotional wellbeing. They
referred to sexist assumptions permeating society as undermining young
women's sense of selfworth – e.g. *Rosemary*: 'because we live in a patriarchal
society . . . males are more valued.' In two ways their comments also reflected
the influence of prominent theories in feminist therapy concerning the
centrality of the mother–daughter relationship as *the* medium through which
the impact of subordination through gender is transmitted. First, they spoke

of women's mothers' emotional needs being paramount. They also commented on fathers seeming to be absent from active emotional engagement with their children (Eichenbaum and Orbach 1984; 1985).

However, a tension between these comments by the counsellors and their other descriptions of women's experience, suggested that the counsellors may have been over generalizing here, perhaps from a commitment to the centrality of the mother–daughter relationship as depicted in writings on feminist therapy. For example, in keeping with women's comments to us, the counsellors described women as being critical of their mother's treatment of them. *Rosemary*: 'The overall feeling that comes across constantly is that mother's love is *insufficient* . . . even though at times they will say, "Well yes, I know my mother did love me really."' The counsellors also described how fathers might provide the more close and sustaining relationship for their children. *Miriam*: 'There are plenty of examples where women will say, "Actually my father was the one who was my mum" . . . and what they mean is that "my father was warm and loving and held me and made me feel I was OK."'

The gendered nature of social relations was also seen as lying at the heart of women's unsatisfactory experience of adult relationships. Thus the counsellors' comments endorsed a major tendency of heterosexual relationships as depicted in women's accounts. *Fran*: 'The key relationship with a man in each case, supposed to give them the central part of their life . . . has brought them unhappiness – a sense of loss of control over their lives . . . subordination to somebody else's definition of them.' The counsellors also identified the sexism women experienced in such relationships as part of the sexism suffusing social relations generally. *Miriam*: 'The unequal opportunity in education and work [has] a huge impact on women and women's mental health . . . because it's almost like they're shifting a huge weight of prejudice against women just by being where they are.'

However, the counsellors' adherence to the explanatory power of ideas of gender subordination also limited their analysis of women's experience. Empirically their observations testified to a capacity for self-expression and assertiveness amongst the most unhappy of women, despite their being subject to gender subordination. In this way their comments confirmed the evidence from women's accounts.

> *Rosemary*: Subordination is the lot of women in our society and girls and women feel it all the time – and this awful sense . . . is one, I think, of *struggle* so what has characterized these relationships is a struggle to be themselves.

However, such observations remained unanalysed; the question mark they raised against a theory of gender subordination being able to account for the state of women's emotional welfare in an all-pervasive way remained unnoticed.

Sexism in therapeutic practice

The counsellors identified the sexism in social relations more generally as also permeating therapeutic practice. In keeping with feminist critiques (see Chapter 1), they were alert to the ways in which women's experience of previous therapeutic care could be stigmatizing and subordinating. They described about 50 per cent of women they saw as having had previous medical or psychiatric intervention, frequently with negative affects. Elspeth spoke at length of a woman who had suffered post-natal depression, had been labelled as depressive, and told that she would have a problem of depression for all of her life.

> *Rosemary*: for a lot of the women, its been terribly conditional. They can only get a certain kind of help if their doctor thinks so, or they saw a psychiatrist and they will say to me almost in surprise, 'Actually I liked her or him and it was quite helpful. But it was only 10 minutes, once every six weeks.'

A further consequence of the counsellors' awareness of sexism in therapeutic practice was their concern that feminist therapy was offered by *women* counsellors. They hoped this would provide some safeguard against sexism. As Heenan (1988) has argued, there is no guarantee that a woman counsellor's approach will be non-sexist. However, there is evidence of generalized assumptions about women's subordination, informing male mental health workers' practice (Barnes and Maple 1992: Ch. 1). Walker's review of research evidence also suggests that although there are instances of women therapists having possibly exploitative sexual relations with male clients; the indications are that male therapists behaving in this way with female clients is far more common (Walker 1990: Ch. 4). Confirmatory evidence of this trend continues to come forward (Mihill 1993). Therefore the counsellors' standpoint may not be misplaced.

The question of empowerment

The counsellors also defined a central aim of feminist therapy as being to empower women. Their standpoint here seemed egalitarian in the following ways. First, they conceptualized empowerment as a process of levelling up women's power, as opposed to women being encouraged to seek power over others.

> *Elspeth*: It's to do with power, but not in terms of power over people, but feeling a powerful person, feeling that I'm OK and that I have a right

to be in the world and have a right to have a say in the world . . . that's very important for women.

Second, in keeping with the self-help spirit informing the growth of feminist therapy more generally (see Chapter 1), the counsellors had tried to even up women's life chances by making better options available. *Fran*, on the Centre: 'It's about showing that there are other ways of treating people who come with emotional distress, other than labelling them and treating them as if they're inhuman . . . we're a drop in the ocean, but we've actually started providing it.'

However, the counsellors' commitment to challenging sexist subordi-nation embodied a strategic limitation. They aimed to rectify the damage to women's emotional welfare incurred through dominating male relations. However, as feminist therapists, they did not aim to engage directly with men at all through workshops or teach-ins. Such strategies would seem to have offered the chance of lifting some of the burden of change off women's shoulders and challenged the idea that women alone were responsible for rectifying their emotional suffering. The counsellors' rejection of such strategies seemed to stem ironically from their determination to provide women with the best opportunity to attain emotional fulfilment. They saw it as essential to protect women from direct contact with the contaminating effects of male power – as women worked to understand it, began to recover from it, and set their own standards for their future wellbeing. This drew their energies to a separatist approach.

Feminist solidarity

Reflecting ideas of feminist solidarity, the counsellors emphasized the importance of drawing on their own personal experience, amongst other things in their work. As women, they saw themselves as having a lot in common with their clients.

> *Elspeth*: What I draw on most at an emotional level, as opposed to an intellectual thing, where I draw obviously mostly on my theory, supervision and practice . . . is to do with my own life. I think more than anything it's knowing what's happened to me.

This approach may have conveyed to women participants that in a major respect, the resources that were going into the work from both parties were on a par with each other. The drawback was that too ready an assumption of parallels between the counsellors' own lives and those of women they worked with could lead the counsellors to gloss over differences of profound importance to the women themselves (Butler and Wintram 1991: 76).

One remaining aspect of the counsellors' feminist perspective is discussed later in the chapter, because it is so inextricably bound up with the detail of practice and organizational strategies. The counsellors saw it as consistent with the aim of equality for women, to be committed to cooperative working relationships both with women clients and amongst themselves.

Awareness of social divisions other than gender

The counsellors acknowledged that women alone did not experience social inequality. *Rosemary*: 'I'm not so daft as to think that the only subordinates in life are women. Elderly, children, blacks, poor – there are dominant subordinate conflicts operating in so many other areas.' They also emphasized that women's inequality did not result solely from the gendered nature of social relations. They commented on how lesbian women welcomed contact with the Centre as one setting in which their sexuality would not be pathologized. *Miriam* also commented on the impact of class on women's emotional wellbeing, 'It's something I feel I've been very aware of as a working-class woman myself, and yet something I don't feel I've got a satisfactory kind of conceptual framework to handle.' She also discussed how she and her colleagues had been helping workers from minority ethnic groups 'to get the skills they need, to do the work they see needs doing . . . some of what they want is . . . to know where they can get training which is going to be some use to them . . . is not intrinsically racist, for example.'

However, the counsellors denied the influence of social divisions apart from gender, any fundamental role in shaping emotional identity and wellbeing. Instead they appealed to the idea of gender's transcending influence.

> *Fran*: The women who are involved here vary from very working-class and materially deprived backgrounds, to well off working-class to actual middle-class parents who were professionals – and that can make a difference to the sense of material deprivation that was experienced by the child – but it makes no difference to the sense of emotional deprivation at all, it's just, it's not a significant variant.

Moreover, there was no discussion of racism or heterosexism as possibly superseding gender as the central focus in practice. Nor did the counsellors or the coordinator comment on disablism or ageism as a specific focus in the work of the Centre. The general perspective on social divisions other than gender that the counsellors seemed to adopt was, therefore, that in certain respects they registered their importance, without seeing them as main foci of practice. In this way their position reflected mainstream feminist practice on psychosocial problems at the time. The impact of social divisions other than gender on women's welfare was acknowledged. However, this was not treated as being of equal or paramount importance (Graham 1992).

Recognition that from a feminist perspective it is important to tackle other dimensions to social inequality than gender, also opens up the possibility of response to men's emotional suffering being a valid feminist project. The counsellors acknowledged that men's wellbeing could be undermined by social inequality. Empirical confirmation of this exists. For example, Barnes and Maple (1992: 11) refer to evidence that women are twice as likely to be taking tranquillizers, and two-thirds of those taking anti-depressants are women. Alternatively this could be expressed as one-third of the population taking tranquillizers and anti-depressants are men. In this respect, Blaxter in her study of the effects of varying levels of income on health found, 'For psycho-social health, low income, independently of social class, increased the likelihood of greater malaise for both men and women of all ages' (Blaxter 1990: 71–2). However, the counsellors – possibly influenced by their separatist stance – and in keeping with a general trend in the practice of feminist therapy, did not tangle with this as an issue for the Centre to pursue.

Putting this issue forward here for consideration is not to disregard the importance of focusing on women's experience or the degree of distress women endure. Instead, it is to acknowledge one dimension to men's experience. Moreover, it is crucial that recognition of sexist behaviour on men's part informs any interventions relating to men's emotional wellbeing. Burstow's discussion of attempting this, reveals just how difficult this may be in practice (1992: Ch. 6).

The counsellors did acknowledge the role of adult–child power differentials in shaping emotional wellbeing. This was implied in Fran's reference to the greater room for manoeuvre which adulthood brings.

> *Fran*: Part of the process of therapy is that [the woman] can see that she doesn't need to go on reacting in the present as though she was still three years old and defined by that situation she was in then, and unable to do anything about it because it's not possible at three; but at 30 or 40 or 50 it's possible.

However, they did not theorize the exercise of adult–child power as a form of social injustice requiring and also being amenable to measures to produce general changes in existing social relations. Their standpoint here reflected their psychotherapeutic perspective, the significance of which is discussed next in detail.

A psychotherapeutic approach

The counsellors' standpoint

The counsellors' approach to psychotherapy did not simply reflect a feminist perspective, i.e. interrogating psychotherapeutic principles and practice on the basis of the extent to which these furthered anti-sexist aims. Instead their adherence to it seemed to derive from their primary commitment to how they defined the role of counsellor/therapist. This was to understand and relieve emotional distress defined in generalized terms, as opposed to suffering brought about by the sexist nature of social relations.

> *Miriam*: I would firstly say I'm there for the client. They're actually coming to me and saying, that, 'I'm in a real mess with this, that, or the other, or I'm hurting terribly, or I'm desperate', and actually my first commitment is to help them find out what that's about and get out of it.

The counsellors seemed to have found that a psychotherapeutic approach had offered both a convincing explanation of the origins of emotional suffering and of a route to freedom involving the efforts of a counsellor; moreover, that it continued to do so. The origins of emotional suffering lay for the most part in personal experience of parent–child relationships in childhood which had invalidated women's feelings of selfworth. Women clients could be helped to understand and face what had happened to undermine their capacity for emotional fulfilment, even if they had not originally been consciously aware of the existence of a causal process or its nature. They could then be helped to renounce what was trapping them emotionally and behave differently, despite these inhibitions possibly still having some power. (For Freud's own summary of psychoanalytic concepts and practice from which these ideas were distilled, see Freud, 1973: part 2.)

The counsellors' adherence to the intricacies of this mode of explanation and intervention was in evidence across all their accounts, but succinctly illustrated in Elspeth's and Fran's.

> *Elspeth*: They're going to dare to look at things . . . that perhaps they have been frightened all their lives to look at. And the aim . . . is to see if they can understand what the discomfort is about. Nearly always it's because the feelings they have are inappropriate for their current situation. So put simply they're behaving as if, all the time, it still matters desperately what they do must please their mother or whatever . . . The beginning part then is to help them to be something that's a mixture of cognitive thought for understanding and observing and, on the other hand, feeling, because unless they feel it, it doesn't have any meaning to them anyway. Then they move from having seen it to letting go of it, the pattern that's been such hell for them. Then, hopefully they move onto the third stage which is trying to do something else, but recognizing the power of the old stuff continually reasserts itself, works in stronger opposition to what they're trying to do that's different, and so to increase all the time this bit of themselves.

> *Fran*: When a client comes she is saying she's in pain, emotional pain, as

opposed to any other sort of pain. The way I understand that pain is that it's about an unconscious unresolved emotional pain . . . a particular pattern of making relationships with a man or with men or with other women, it may be sexual or non-sexual, it depends sort of on what area of their life this occurs in . . . a repeated pattern which is not doing her any good and causing her a lot of distress and usually people have gone through this several times before they get to us, but by then they know there's something they want to sort out. So – I would see my work . . . as about finding out the sources of this unresolved conflict or pain, and trying to help the woman resolve what that first difficulty was about before, to remove the pain, so that she no longer needs to go on repeating it.

The main implications of the counsellors' psychotherapeutic standpoint

The main implications for intervention of this standpoint were threefold. First, it focused attention on the power of earlier interpersonal interaction to create self-identity, through children's introjection of the value adults had placed on them. Second, it played down the power of contemporary interpersonal and social relations in adulthood in undermining emotional wellbeing. Third, it emphasized an individual's capacity to shape their emotional wellbeing in adulthood and the importance of assuming responsibility for doing so. In different ways all these implications were problematic for taking account of the need to tackle profound social inequalities, in order to foster emotional wellbeing.

First, concentrating on the effects of childhood relationships meant that the counsellors were attuned to what was the site of a great deal of the unhappiness women had experienced – as described in their accounts. In this respect therefore, women's emotional needs were unlikely to be subordinated yet again, this time in the course of feminist therapy. Such an approach also meant that the counsellors were sensitive to the effects of the unequal power relations that children underwent, as an important dimension to experience. However, because they did not theorize such unequal power relations as reflecting widespread social conditions requiring widespread changes to ameliorate them, their findings remained within the universe of therapy. The findings were considered and dealt with solely on an individual basis – rather than being transmitted into public debate as subject matter indicating the need for profound and extensive social change.

Perhaps this conservative approach on the counsellors' part was fuelled by Freudian ideas that relationships rooted in parental power as the mainspring of individual development were part of the natural order. Therefore, they were unchanging and, by inference, unchangeable through preventative action. For example:

> a still higher degree of interest must attach to the influence of a situation which every child is destined to pass through and which follows inevitably from the factor of the prolonged period during which a child is cared for by other people and lives with his parents. I am thinking of the Oedipus complex.

> (Freud 1973:44)

A further upshot of the counsellors holding this viewpoint was that theoretically it was difficult for them to account for instances of children experiencing comparative freedom from parental influence. Moreover, it was difficult for them to draw lessons from this, of preventative measures that might be used to even up children's experience of comparative powerlessness.

The second consequence of concentrating on the power of earlier interpersonal interaction to undermine self-identity, was the marginalization of the undermining effect of experience of social divisions in adulthood. Women's accounts had suggested that undermining as the legacy of childhood relationships could be, the destructive power of adult relationships in their own right could match this. The counsellors acknowledged the impact of events subsequent to childhood. They also showed that they were aware of the effects of gender being intertwined in young women's experience. For example, they frequently commented on how boy children were elevated as important in parent's eyes and girl children allotted caring roles against their own interests. Yet when illustrating the form that the aetiology of emotional suffering took, the counsellors, as in Elspeth and Fran's accounts, unfailingly returned to client's childhoods as their starting point. Such an emphasis on individual personal development in childhood as crucial to the aetiology of emotional problems obscured the potential of current sexist social relations to have an equally powerful effect in undermining women's emotional wellbeing. By extension it also obscured the potential of other social divisions affecting adults to do so. Thus, the counsellors' adherence to a psychotherapeutic approach detracted from their feminism and also possibly limited the account they took of the effects of a range of other forms of social inequality in adult life.

Finally, the counsellors did not hold a facile view of the strength of countervailing forces ranged against people's emotional wellbeing. They did not talk as though therapy could result in an utterly happy existence. Nevertheless, the emphasis on the key to emotional wellbeing in adulthood lying in the individual's capacity to shape it, once they had come to terms with emotional impediments derived from childhood, ran a twofold risk of playing down the scale of effort required to counteract the undermining effects on emotional wellbeing of inequality permeating society. First, it obscured the need for extensive collective action to make any impression on contemporary inequalities in social relations – both a consistent theme and lesson from the contemporary women's movement (Rowbotham 1989). Second, it did not take account of how it might justly not be regarded as the lone responsibility of the individuals adversely affected by forms of social inequality to carry out such work (Dominelli 1988). In this last respect the counsellors' psychotherapeutic standpoint compounded some shortcomings of their separatist feminist approach.

A commitment to counselling

Features in common with psychotherapy

The counsellors' accounts suggested that they regarded the theory and practice of 'counselling' and 'psychotherapy' as interpenetrating each other. For example, while they all drew on psychotherapeutic concepts, they also all typified their work as counselling. *Rosemary*, on her work prior to that at the Centre:

> at [the contraceptive advice centre] I convened the counselling team because of what we found there . . . you would read the medical notes and it would say everybody was all right, because the only thing that was asked was, 'How were you coping on the pill', but in fact some of these women had terrible problems, but they never described them or talked about them . . .

Two of the distinctive tenets of counselling specifically identified by the counsellors as reference points for their practice are also present in psychotherapeutic practice: the idea of being non-judgemental in interaction with clients and the idea of being non-directive (Truax and Carkhuff 1975: Ch. 2). Both approaches were also subscribed to by the counsellors on the basis that they would help to counteract the undermining effect of past relationships on women's present self-esteem, in the interests of women subsequently seeking a better emotional deal for themselves. Moreover, in referring to the origins of the emotional problems that required such approaches, the counsellors echoed psychotherapeutic concepts of possibly unconscious impediments to emotional wellbeing acquired in childhood.

> *Elspeth*: being non-judgemental, as it were, enables them [the women] gradually to perhaps be less judgemental, with themselves, and so allowing themselves to see these – psychological blocks, much more clearly.

Then discussing the purpose of a non-directive approach:

> *Elspeth*: They've learned to be dependent upon adults. So they're

looking to you for solutions – and its only when they start to solve their own problems then the thing starts to change.

Counselling in contrast to psychotherapy

As they discussed counselling, the counsellors did not seem to play down the need for other forms of social change to occur, as had been the case when they had focused on a psychotherapeutic approach in their work. Instead, they seemed to conceptualize the relationship of counselling to the wider social context. They saw it as being one means of encouraging women as individuals to obtain conditions more conducive to their emotional wellbeing, while the women concerned might still be trapped in broader social conditions which they could do little to change.

> *Elspeth*: What it is, is to actually help somebody feel good about themselves ... Often you know ... women will compromise enormously ... They can't leave the relationship probably mainly because of their children, but [also] their financial dependence ... But what they can do, sometimes, is to actually feel less put down by it and so they may take more time to themselves, you know by coming to a group or doing other things in their lives.

There are two problems with this approach. First, it begs the question of whether, if as individuals women participated in collective action, they might not be able to produce more widespread change in their interests. Second, it seems likely to support the continuation of the status quo, thereby possibly contributing to women's present and future emotional wellbeing being undermined.

Non-hierarchical forms of practice?

Introduction

The degree to which theoretical perspectives commonly employed in feminist therapy take account of the need to tackle profound social inequalities and can therefore be considered egalitarian has been reviewed through the counsellors' accounts. Now the question is addressed of whether or not counsellor–client interaction in feminist therapy simply replicates the subordinating nature of other relationships which women experience as undermining their emotional wellbeing. The fuller answer to this question obviously needs to draw on women participants' experience. Evidence is taken from counsellors' accounts about how hierarchical the power relations running through counsellor–client interaction are and the significance of this for the emotional wellbeing of the women clients.

The state of debate about the power relationship between the counsellor and client in feminist therapy is problematic. First, there tends to be a separation between discussion of what feminist therapy aims to do – based on counsellors' anecdotal evidence, and references to the question of whether or not counsellors do behave in a dominating way (e.g. Chaplin 1988; Walker 1990). This separation enables examination of the outcomes of feminist therapy to slide away from the question of whether the behaviour of counsellors in practice undermines the non-hierarchical aims of their work. It also draws attention away from just how hard it may be to adhere to such aims. If counsellors' behaviour is less than perfect here, it does not differ from feminist practice more generally. The argument that the egalitarian ends of feminist activism should be prefigured by the creation of egalitarian social relations within feminist initiatives has been well rehearsed. However, the idealism embodied in this approach has also been chronicled as accompanied by more suspect assumptions and practices resulting from the influence of the unequal social relations that feminists set out to combat (Langan and Day 1992).

Second, when the power relations between counsellor–client in feminist therapy *are* discussed, the mode of debate is unsatisfactory. There are exhortations that such a relationship should be egalitarian, e.g. Chaplin, 'the counsellor is not there to dominate or have power over the client' (1988: 7). There are assumptions that this is the case: 'The approach is egalitarian with a careful avoidance of the one-down position' (Penfold and Walker 1984: 233). Alternatively there are counter assumptions that as therapist–client encounters are innately hierarchical, by definition those in feminist therapy, as a form of therapy, must be so (Ussher 1991).

To compensate for these shortcomings in current debate, here analysis of counsellor–client power relations is integrated with analysis of practice in feminist therapy. This is done by focusing on the extent to which interactions between counsellor and client are hierarchical in practice, and the significance for women's emotional welfare of this.

Recognition of women's psychological strengths

The counsellors' glowing accounts of the personal strengths women brought into therapy suggested that once women engaged in feminist therapy, their self-esteem would not be undermined by their being treated as though they were psychologically inadequate.

> *Elspeth*: They're saying they haven't got the psychological strength, that doesn't mean they're psychologically weak, but we're, that is society, asking them to do superhuman tasks . . . so to suggest they might give up some of the superhuman tasks is how we're [the counsellors] asking them to cope . . .

The counsellors' comments on what women gained from feminist therapy were also consistent with a non-psychopathologizing approach to the resources they brought. For example, *Fran* commented on: 'seeing them becoming less self-critical, less harsh on themselves, less expecting themselves to be perfect, or more realistic about their real potential'. The theme of the strengths women brought into therapy was maintained in the counsellors' description of women's motivation for coming. Here, the counsellors' views concurred with the picture women had given as opposed to the picture provided by some theoretical tendencies in feminist therapy (see discussion in Chapter 3). The counsellors did not depict women as cowed into psychological passivity. Instead, their descriptions recognized women's capacity for self-expression and assertiveness: how women were unhappy about and critical of the state they were in and trying – even if apparently against all the odds, to do something about it.

> *Fran*: Some of them are actually desperate, a real sense of desperation about how awful they feel about themselves. And an awareness somewhere that it doesn't have to be like that . . . they want to be able to have satisfying relationships . . . They want to be able to feel free to use this potential they have, to study, or work or voluntary work, whatever they choose . . . an enormously strong motivation.

The counsellors also valued a further aspect of the resources women brought into feminist therapy – support from friends. The counsellors did not disparage friendship's contribution to women's emotional wellbeing as somehow inferior to feminist therapy. Instead, echoing women's accounts, they recognized its central importance, but as providing a different form of support with its own limitations, imposed by its own conventions.

> *Miriam*: Most women who come here . . . say that one of the reasons that brings them is that their friendship network can no longer give them [the support] they need . . . Many . . . say 'I wouldn't be able to go on if it wasn't for my friend, but the thing is that it's not helping me resolve the problem.'

Despite this positive valuation of the resources women brought into feminist therapy, the counsellors' accounts suggested that in two ways they also adopted a subordinating approach which was problematic for the wellbeing of women participants. First, by using criteria for selection as a means of control, and second, by making assumptions about the superiority of their input – compared with that of women participants – for bringing about change. These two negative facets of the counsellors' practice are discussed next. In both, elitist assumptions attaching to the professional role they had assumed are apparent.

Criteria for selection as a means of control

The counsellors accepted only self-referrals. They were adamant that women were sufficiently expert on their problems not to need a professional to refer them. However, the principles on which the counsellors and coordinator organized women's access to counselling at the Centre provided evidence that they exercised power over women, with questionable consequences.

The counsellors' rationale for their approach was to make the most of certain skills they held. The numbers wanting feminist therapy far exceeded those that could be taken on by the counsellors directly, given the personnel the Centre's funding could support. Therefore, some rationing procedure had to operate. However, the counsellors did not operate a procedure of strict rotation. The ultimate and, therefore, primary determinant of whether or not women received counselling after contacting the Centre, was how well they met the counsellors' criteria of suitability for engaging in psychotherapy. In this way not only did control of access to help remain firmly in the counsellors' hands, but also the process institutionalized the theoretical primacy of psychotherapy.

The coordinator's policy was also in keeping with this. She offered an assessment interview when women wanted counselling as a result of generalized and/or acute emotional distress, or particularly referred to the problem as originating in childhood. On the basis of this interview the following outcomes were possible – short or long-term one-to-one counselling; group work; a place on the waiting list; if the waiting list was closed – advice re other resources; or the assessment interview itself would stand as a piece of work.

The counsellors' concern not to waste anyone's time by embarking on interventions for which they lacked expertise was understandable. Nevertheless, there was a strong air of the 'client' fitting the service, rather than vice versa, in the counsellors' collective account of the most important criteria informing their decision to work with someone.

Q What criteria did you use for taking on women?
A That it was 'the kind of problem that it would be possible to resolve or improve by psychotherapy – (i.e. to do with severe conflict over relationships or how the person perceived themselves, or feelings they felt overwhelmed by, such as physical ailments with large psychological component).

Example – A woman in her fifties who had previously been hospitalized for a 'severe obsessional neurosis' and who came to the Centre. She was unable to leave her home or travel anywhere alone, and her life dominated by ritualistic behaviour. She had a long history of being battered as a child and as a wife.

Even greater store was set by whether or not women were willing and able to cooperate in what was viewed as the psychotherapeutic process

> This criteria would be given the greatest importance – assessment of some way in which the client provided evidence that she experienced the initial interview therapeutically i.e. was able to talk enough, listen enough, share thinking and move on to see the relevance for herself of the therapy process in relation to her problem. This would show, for example in her recognizing something she had not been aware of before, such as a pattern in her life that gives her pain which she feels compelled to repeat . . . This criteria is most essential because it gives both therapist and client a joint experience of the process about which a decision has to be made.
> (Collective statement by the counsellors on the criteria they employed
> for accepting women for therapy)

There were several drawbacks to this approach. First, it was inequitable. Some women might have equally serious emotional needs as those selected, but the insights and methods of psychotherapy might not be relevant. Second, previous discussion of the counsellors' psychotherapeutic tenets suggested that these could not be seen as offering a comprehensive definition of the emotional problems women faced. This concentration on psychotherapy was therefore likely to lead to their work being irrelevant to important aspects of women's experience, even if they gained a place. The following criteria referred to by the counsellors, also exposed the inequity of their only being prepared to tackle emotional distress originating in certain ways. They were not prepared to take on women experiencing acute material distress – 'Assessment of the clients' support systems i.e. partners, family, friends, etc. during the process of therapy . . . If the client's practical problems i.e. homelessness are at crisis point, psychotherapy would not be perceived as relevant' (collective statement by the counsellors).

The 'superiority' of the counsellors' input

The counsellors may have valued the emotional resources women brought to feminist therapy. They also acknowledged that, in the final analysis, the initiative to decide whether or not to embark on changes in perception or activity lay with the women. *Elspeth*: 'Ultimately the power to change lies with the client, of course.' However, the counsellors seemed to rate their own contribution as even more powerful than that of women participants in terms of the means it provided to bring about change. *Miriam* on the counsellor–client relationship: 'It's unequal because she doesn't have, in a sense, the skills such as I have and we, she is, we are using for her benefit.' In fairness to the counsellors – from their comments – such a belief in their powers was also heavily reinforced by women attributing healing powers to them. Elspeth commented on feeling under pressure from clients to exercise superior powers to solve their problems – as they turned their 'large appealing eyes' on her she felt somehow she had to 'come up with the goods'.

Some commentators on feminist therapy have argued that it is because of feminist therapy's placebo effect that the client benefits. 'The therapist is able to exert influence because of the client's need for change, expectation that the therapist has the necessary resources for that change, and the power attributed to the therapist' (Dworkin 1984: 305). The drawback to a situation where counsellors' powers are regarded as superior is that it perpetuates the idea that the power to determine women's emotional wellbeing lies or should lie with others. As a result, women may encourage themselves or be encouraged simply to exchange their parents' or partner's prescriptions for their emotional wellbeing for the therapist's. The outcome is that they are then no nearer to exercising their own capacity to define and express their emotional needs.

The counsellors could not be held accountable for women ascribing to the ideology that those involved as professionals in the relief of suffering had superior powers (Miles 1988). But knowing of this danger, were the counsellors' efforts to put their resources at the disposal of women, but within what was identified as a counselling relationship, enough? *Elspeth* raised this awkward point:

> I think the client will always invest power, of course, in the counsellor, and so what we have to question here is whether we are perpetrating the whole sort of power syndrome.

Counsellors could have confined their activities to promoting co-counselling or self-help counselling group initiatives amongst women. The idea that self-help groups (Butler and Wintram 1991) and co-counselling (Jackins 1978, Ernst and Goodison 1981) share in common, is that all the parties involved both contribute to and gain from encouragement to address and resolve emotional problems they face. This is as opposed to unchanging specialist counsellor/client roles where the counsellor and the client both contribute, but in the interests of the client's improved emotional wellbeing. Co-counselling or self-help groups do not necessarily guarantee equivalence of status or power (see respectively Ernst and Goodison 1981: 51 and Butler and Wintram, 1991). Nevertheless, the counsellors did not put forward substituting a co-counselling model for their role as a possible solution to the problem. This may have reflected a determination to safeguard their role, or they may have been imbued with the idea of the importance of professional counselling skills. It could also have been – as they alluded to in their discussion of friendship – because they thought that some women needed one relationship, where for once, they could concentrate on their own needs alone.

The counsellors *had* participated in promoting self-help groups and also commented very enthusiastically on the opportunity they provided for women's own counselling skills to develop. *Fran*: 'There was something about that sense of sharing and affirmation from other women . . . the effect of it was multiplication, not addition, it was quite boggling, so I think groups are tremendously powerful.'

As a collective, the counsellors and coordinator also promoted a pro-gramme of workshops involving group work on a wide range of issues, such as assertiveness training and life-planning skills. Most were run by pro-fessional trainers, but they incorporated the identification of common problems or interests by the women participants and self-help groups.

However, while in parts of their practice at the Centre the counsellors were happy to move some or all of the way to a self-help ideology, there was also some evidence of counsellors valuing the more dominating position over women clients that one-to-one work could offer. In comparing groupwork and one-to-one work Rosemary revealed that the one-to-one session was seen as enabling the counsellor to exert more leverage on a woman.

> *Rosemary*: I don't think it's [group work] all much different except that you're working with the interactions of the person who's talking at the time and the others as well as yourself. So in a way it's much more difficult, yet in another way you've got a very interesting additional element coming in . . . of course, it's [group work] all so much more broken up because if you work on one woman you can be darn sure you're not going to work on her again for a week, whereas the one-to-one stuff she comes back for it again and again . . .

Then, acknowledging some 'patient non-compliance':

> I mean you may say it works both ways that in a way, that's so panic stricken making for some people they then cancel the next appointment or they come half an hour late or something.

Women's desperation, compounded by the counsellors' assumption of the superiority of their skills may therefore have contributed to feminist therapy being a situation where yet again women were in danger of having their emotional resources treated in a subordinating way. However, the real culprit was the dire nature of social relations generally in women's lives. These left them desperate to seek out a means of obtaining a better emotional state and therefore primed to identify what therapists offered, as a power greater than theirs.

> *Miriam*: there's the possibility of, for example getting out of years of agony and pain, and for many clients it feels like a matter of life and death, they often say things like, with a great deal of shame . . . for a long

time they haven't wanted to live or they've lived because they believe suicide is wrong or bad, but really they don't want to live.

Counsellors as 'emotional midwives'

The saving grace in a situation where the reinforcement of the status of professional identity seemed to threaten the chances of co-working being a reality, seemed to lie in the counsellor's determined attempt to put what was defined as a superior source of power – their skills – at the disposal of clients. Counsellors aimed to act as 'emotional midwives', i.e. to be the means at women's disposal to facilitate their efforts at bringing about their own emotional liberation. The high degree of commitment among the counsellors and the coordinator to creating such a form of interaction is demonstrated in its consistency as a theme in describing the aims of their work. It emerged in the coordinator's brief account of an example of her best work.

> I think my best efforts were talking to a client of Elspeth's who phoned up ... she was very flat, depressed, and just talking about nothing serious or deep, she changed in the period she was on the phone, 20 minutes to half an hour. She began to get brighter ... She doesn't always need a lot of time. Sometimes if somebody knows it's available, they don't need to use it. Perhaps they have an internal conversation.

It was also reflected in counsellors' accounts of examples of their worst work. In different and, at times, dramatic ways they described how they felt they had been falling down on the job when their own state or preoccupations had got in the way of concentrating on what the client needed to aim at.

> *Rosemary*: Last week I was really ill. And I went through a terrible interview with somebody and five minutes after they left I was vomiting like mad, I had a dreadful migraine. In the interview I knew I wasn't even really there, for this person and I know, looking back on it, what I should have said was, 'Look, I'm too ill', in fact I wrote to them afterwards and said, 'Please let's strike that out and don't count it as an interview.' I was just holding on to myself every minute to get through and I thought afterwards, 'What the hell made me do that? What a silly thing to do', but they'd come rather a long way, and ... what I learned from it is how important it is to be available in an interview with your own stuff well tucked away.

Fran's account of an example of her best efforts is quoted at length to set out the positive nature of the process of emotional midwifery as described by the counsellors.

> *Fran*: This is a woman where I suspect her own mother had an incestuous relationship with *her* father but certainly what she's passed

on to the woman who's my client is, a very very, the most fundamentally, deep distrust of men, 'You can't trust men', is one message and the other message is, 'You can't trust men around children.' So that this led the woman who's my client in fact not to have a child until her marriage was actually on the rocks and she knew she was splitting up from her husband and then knowing she was going to be a single parent she went ahead and got pregnant. So these messages from her mother have determined what she could do in her life in very, very fundamental ways.

And this mother was extremely unavailable to her, they never had any physical contact, she could never talk to her mother, her mother was always, she always worked and was always busy in the kitchen, so that if ever she wanted her mother she had to go and seek her, the mother wouldn't really communicate with her. She, the girl was an only child and she was given everything materially so she was bought off materially. There was no emotional contact at all and no physical contact.

This woman has kept in daily contact with her mother and hadn't been able to get through to any feelings about how she actually felt about her mother, she could narrate instances, and say intellectually how it was, but she wasn't getting through to anything about actual feeling about her mother . . .

What I decided to do, which is most unusual for me was to try something from Gestalt, [See Note 1 at end of chapter] with this woman – and I did this out of the blue with no warning and I moved from my chair and said, 'Your mother is on that chair, what would you like to say to her?', because she'd arrived feeling het up about her mother that day and she couldn't say anything to her – so I said 'Right, you've obviously got a block, something's blocking you saying what you want to say to your mother, so we'll put the block on the chair, what do you want to say to the block?' – and she then started what must have gone on for 15 or 20 minutes of shouting and sobbing and getting out through gratingly gritted teeth how much she hated her mother, hated all that she had done to her, hated her never loving her, hated her mother determining everything of the way she could be in her life – and as I say, this went for a long time and at the end she was absolutely exhausted and she got a sore throat, 'cause it had hurt her so much getting it all out – and I was sitting next to her with my arm round her, encouraging her, she was just sobbing, and sobbing and sobbing.

And for me that was important – and feels like a reasonable piece of work, because it was about this woman getting in touch with how she really felt about this woman who was her mother, actually working on an emotional level at this block. And it was obviously important for her because what happened subsequently is, for the very first time, she's actually been able to feel herself as separate from her mother. And know that when her mother, her mother for instance has really been getting at her about her current man friend and her plans to go on holiday with him, and she actually is not affected by this because she knows it's her mother talking about her own issues, her own material, not hers, the daughter's . . . So for the first time she's actually able to make some decisions in her life about her relationship with a man and letting this man near to her child.

The configuration of power relations between counsellor and client described here seems crucial to feminist therapy having a liberating effect on women's emotional welfare. The interaction between counsellor and women client amounted to the antithesis of the hierarchical relationships which women had described as undermining their emotional wellbeing and held great similarities to relationships which had helped to restore it (see Chapters 2 and 3).

In the emotional midwifery depicted in Fran's account, the other party to the relationship, the counsellor, employed their intellectual, emotional, physical/material resources in a way which valued as opposed to subordinated the woman's need for affection and capacity to express it. As a result, in such interaction the woman had the rare opportunity to have these requirements met. As this happened, the lie was also given to the woman's persona being the cause of her unhappiness. In the interaction with the counsellor, she lived through a demonstration that once the hierarchical nature of the social relations she was caught up in was changed, so her emotional difficulties were diminished. She was given a chance to be 'more herself'. The further consequence of this was an increase in her feelings of selfworth.

The experience of feminist therapy described here may have promoted the emotional wellbeing of the individual woman concerned. However, the account also echoed short-comings in the counsellors' theoretical perspectives which hold problematic consequences for women's and others' wellbeing more generally, and which also need to be checked out in the women's accounts. First, focusing exclusively on women in therapy as subordinated, might lead to disregarding the issue of the extent to which their behaviour subverts the interests of others. Second, concentrating on changes in women's perceptions and subsequent actions as the key to future wellbeing seems to obviate the need for those whose behaviour was or is subordinating to the women to change. Third, concentrating on the undermining effects of women's developmental history, and the operation of gender – as in Fran's account – might marginalize attention to the undermining effects of other dimensions of inequality, such as the impact of relative poverty thereby rendering therapeutic interaction less helpful or irrelevant to women's needs.

Fourth, individuals in the women's lives may have administered subordinating treatment – as in Fran's example – the woman's mother. But at the same time they may also have been the victims of the effects of unequal social relations. Their behaviour may have been driven by their own subordinating experience of inequality – in this case the mother's own experience of sexual abuse. If, in feminist therapy, only the client is conceptualized as a victim, this may lead to pathologizing others in a way that is unjust (Knowles and Cole 1990). Finally, identifying the woman in therapy, alone, as the victim may also lead to perpetuating an unrealistic underestimation of the power of unequal social relations, to subvert emotional wellbeing more generally. The corollary to this is that an inflated idea is conveyed of what therapy may achieve.

Forms of organization – effects on women participants

Introduction

Underpinning and informing interaction between the counsellors and women coming to the Centre were the characteristic forms of its organization. These had features in common with feminist initiatives more generally. Therefore, useful lessons can be drawn from the extent to which they represented a model of equity – in relation to the needs of women participants and in relation to the needs of counsellors and coordinators as workers.

Accessibility

As in most feminist initiatives, the Centre achieved a qualified degree of success in ensuring its accessibility as an organization, to women in differing social circumstances. Counselling was free. Although the amount of funding produced low salaries and modest organizational resources, the counsellors did not consider payment as an option. Therefore, size of income was not an issue in terms of paying fees.

The counsellors and coordinator also tried to cultivate an informal hospitable atmosphere in the Centre. They were anxious to escape the ambience of medical and mental health settings generally, which they saw as conveying the impression of a hierarchy, with the patient at the bottom. Facilities for making hot drinks were readily and always available. Throughout our contact with the Centre, which included dropping in informally and at short notice, we were both impressed by the unhurried, calm atmosphere, whatever the demands on the workers. The coordinator also seemed genuinely interested in the welfare of callers at the Centre or over the phone and did not simply occupy a gatekeeping role.

The premises obtained from the City Council comprised a small, ground floor maisonette in a bleak development. Nevertheless, with minimal material resources, the interior had been transformed. The decor was soothing and attractive – the antithesis of clinical, and the three counselling rooms were furnished with comfortable chairs and floor cushions.

However, the premises did not have wheelchair access. Facilities for women with hearing impairment were not available. A visiting counselling service was not a routine option. Therefore, women who were housebound were not catered for. Issues such as help with fares and the difficulty of arranging childcare, which might have had a bearing on access, were also not addressed. It is only fair to add that assistance with these was beyond the Centre's material resources.

Open-ended time limits

The counsellors also aimed to reverse what they saw as the common pattern where women themselves, or others relating to them or treating them, tended not to give adequate time to meeting women's emotional needs. Instead, at the Centre, counselling and therapy would take as long as it took. Contact would be terminated not on the say-so of the counsellor, or on the basis of a predetermined schedule to fit the Centre's resources, but when the woman concerned decided it was appropriate. The depth of the counsellors' commitment is reflected in Fran's comment, 'My understanding is that actually that's the only way you can work.' The practice may also have owed something to the counsellors' psychotherapeutic approach. Psychotherapy is renowned for running across many years, in some cases, and as such is seen as a lengthy process. Meanwhile, there has been a long-running debate about the advantages of shorter time limited periods of intervention – a few weeks or few months. The argument is that a defined brief period of time for work produces better results because it concentrates the attention and energies of the worker and client and is more manageable by the client (Reid and Epstein 1977; Nelson-Jones 1988; Laws 1991; Kareem and Littlewood 1992).

The acid test of this approach lies in women participants' comments. However, in the context of women's accounts of relationships in childhood and adulthood (Chapters 2 and 3) the length of time spent in counselling and therapy was not that great. Against a background in some cases of a whole lifetime with apparently barely anyone's time and attention devoted to a particular woman's emotional wellbeing, six months counselling at the rate of an hour weekly amounted to just 24 hours. *Elspeth*: 'one hour a week is hardly anything.'

Nevertheless, the counsellors' resources, as personnel, were slender. The counsellors averaged 12 sessions each a week, including assessment interviews. Therefore, the decision to opt for unlimited contact was likely to represent a proportionately substantial reduction in numbers of women who could actually be seen. For example, if all women were routinely seen for three months at a time, the annual turnover would run at something like 144. If three-quarters of the women were seen for at least a year and the rest for three-month periods then the annual turnover would run at something like 63.

By the time we were interviewing, the waiting list for counselling and therapy following initial interviews had been closed due to pressure of demand leading to unconscionable delays. However, the rate at which women were contacting the Centre indicated that the nub of the shortfall was not the way of working which the counsellors' chose. Instead, the general demand from women for what the Centre offered, reflecting women's unmet emotional need and the limited nature of the resources central and local government funding had made available to meet it, was the root of the problem. The coordinator's log of initial contacts with the Centre across a six-month period indicated that excluding contacts clearly seeking information, or appropriately referred on to other more specialized agencies, e.g. centres for psychosexual counselling for couples, the Centre was attracting potential candidates for counselling at an average rate of eight per week, or 192 across six months or 384 in a year. On the basis of these figures, even if counsellors had struck rigidly to a three-month timespan for each woman, there would still have been nearly twice as many women who could not be seen as those who could.

Feedback

The counsellors were very resistant to the idea that their own work could harm people. It was as though they were so committed to helping women and relieving emotional distress that this was an unbearable thought.

> *Elspeth*: It's up to us to make sure they're [the women] not harmed . . . I actually think that people can protect themselves against everything – especially if they are damaged, they've learned to protect themselves.

Apart from this, the counsellors accepted that counselling or therapy generally could damage women. *Rosemary* on her own experience in analysis, 'You can have a sensation that you are owned, that you have lost yourself, that you can't do anything except the therapist says, a sort of massive takeover.' The counsellors also had a critical approach to evidence of the outcomes of their work. They had agreed to the independent assessment represented by our study and had instituted a means of systematic feedback. Follow-up forms were sent out to women six months after they had finished. From these the counsellors hoped to get an indication of women's experience of counselling and whether or not any positive effects were still continuing. They were also alert to the dangers of oversimplification in evaluation: that it might be difficult to disentangle the effects of feminist therapy as one among all the different factors operating in women's lives. *Miriam*: 'But ultimately how do you know, how do you ever know? It's like the stone that's dropped in the pool.'

Absence of collective representation

Despite provisions for individual evaluation, there were none for women participants' collective representation in the running of the Centre. The counsellors and coordinator expressed the view that women picked up the cooperative, non-hierarchical organization of the workers as an indication of the Centre's egalitarian approach. *Bridget*: 'Because it's not hierarchical. That must have an effect.' *Elspeth*: 'They see and feel, I think, the vibes that are here . . . the fact that there isn't a hierarchy.' In this way the Centre's staff fell into the trap of dogmatically identifying certain organizational forms as inherently feminist and thereby egalitarian (Sturdy 1987). Priding themselves on their collective self-management as workers as being in keeping with feminist principles, they failed to see that such an arrangement might need to be extended to include clients, if the whole organization was to be more truly non-hierarchical.

Forms of organization – effects on the counsellors and coordinator

The multiple demands of the work

The counsellors and coordinator saw themselves as benefiting from their work in various ways in their personal life.

> *Elspeth*: Setting up this Centre, it was like my life force really and everything else became second . . . its validated my existence.

Nevertheless, they also admitted that working at the Centre made considerable emotional demands.

> *Rosemary*: The thing that I know always gets at me like stink is when women are suicidal . . . you put your hand out and you can't just hold on to them, they've got to do some holding on to you and if they let go, they do go down the cliff face and you can't go down with them . . . sometimes I find the demands very great and I go home feeling shattered, utterly exhausted.

Such demands also had an impact on their other relationships. *Miriam*: 'A lot of my anxieties . . . and conflicts get dumped at home.'

Material problems compounded the emotional demands of the work. Shoestring financing has been a feature of feminist collectives, as repeatedly the only available funding has been short-term local or central government grants (Gelb 1990). The Centre's funding had followed this pattern. Their Inner City partnership grant was modest. This meant that albeit for a part-time week of 17 hours or pro rata, the counsellors' pay averaged between £3,000 and £3,500 p.a. (The coordinator earned £4,600 p.a. for a 30 hour week.) These salaries compared with £14,240 p.a. full-time pay for social workers in middle management which the counsellors' experience and training would have enabled them to command (personal communication). The stress such a situation can produce – including the difficulty of surviving independently without plunging into poverty, is reflected in *Miriam*'s comments:

> If my relationship broke up I couldn't survive financially, I'd have to sell my flat . . . if I had aspirations to earn a lot of money I would have taken a very different track – but I'm beginning to think you don't have to be poor to do good work . . . I want to be able to pay my electricity bill and hold my end up.

Getting the Centre established, publicizing its activities, developing its range of work and pursuing long-term funding – in addition to day-to-day work, also produced a very demanding all round work load way beyond part-time hours. We observed this in operation. It was also reflected in all the counsellor's comments but epitomized in *Rosemary*'s 'It occupies a very large amount of my life.' These demands were also being juggled with the demands on the counsellors and coordinator as partners and mothers. Their comments indicated that in many respects their male partners were supportive, e.g. Rosemary when contemplating life without her partner.

> *Rosemary*: I've often thought if I had to go back to a totally empty house and nobody to talk to and nobody there . . . I don't know whether I would be able to go on working as a therapist. I hope I would . . . in due course, but I think it makes you very vulnerable.

The counsellors also commented on their older children as being supportive. But despite such support, their comments highlighted the unremitting pressures on women attempting to combine employment with primary responsibility for childcare (Calvert 1985).

> *Fran* (with four children): I know that when I'm rushing out of the Centre at 2.30 and I've got to be at the school gate at 3.30 I'm not really there at the school gate, part of me is still back at work in the last interview or whatever – I'm finding that hard still . . . when I get outside and I discover how much of my personal resources its depleted

. . . when I'm required to give and give and give to the children all evening.

The counsellors' accounts also revealed the risks which a high level of commitment to their work could produce in terms of their male partner's intolerance. The counsellors' experience thus replicated a pattern identified as common amongst women, i.e. the threat of withdrawal of emotional support from male partners acting as a brake on their activism (Curno, et al. 1982). As one counsellor commented:

it really came almost earlier on this year . . . to an absolute crisis in my relationship, in which my partner felt that I put my work first to the extent that I actually didn't want a relationship at all, and that I was working much too much . . . outside Centre hours.

Cooperative working arrangements

In the face of these overall demands how did the aim of establishing collective non-hierarchical ways of working stand up? To what extent did the counsellors' and coordinator's comments suggest they were able to create an equitable division of labour which they found personally supportive?

The counsellors and coordinator appreciated the formative stage of development of their attempts to work non-hierarchically. They were aware that working in this way was against the grain of conventional working experience.

Elspeth: At times I'm sure everybody in the collective has felt they are actually carrying the Centre . . . 'I am responsible for the Centre and if I don't do this, this and this then it's all going to collapse.' I'm learning to feel less of that and I'm sure that's to do with having always worked in a hierarchical situation.

The counsellors commented as well on the demands the attempt to work non-hierarchically made in its own right: for instance, the seemingly slow process of collective decision making. *Rosemary*: 'Speed, speed! it's so damn slow because you have to carry everybody, and feel happy about everybody and look after everybody's feelings and so on.'

The counsellors' and coordinator's comments also demonstrated that allegiance to the ideal of non-hierarchical relations and attempts to implement them could not guarantee their existence. To some extent this was acknowledged. *Miriam*: 'I think that the hierarchies that exist are often to do with having more experience and have more to do with self-ranking, in a way.' However, in common with other feminist enterprises, divisions in society more generally seeped into their working relations (Hudson 1989). For example, the counsellors were adamant that there was no hierarchy of skills. *Rosemary*: 'Bridget [the coordinator] here – she's doing a different job, but she's in no way fundamentally *valued* less.' Nevertheless, at several points the coordinator indicated that she felt in a comparatively isolated, lower status position because of her educational, social and employment background. While describing the organization as 'definitely collective' she added:

> some people are more assertive, more able to put their point of view and I don't find that easy at all – I'm quite frightened of dealing with controversial views. I think that's something to do with the fact I'm the only person who answered an advert to work here . . . and that feels somehow different . . . my coming here is because it's a job. And they can't say that in the same way because of the commitment they had before.

Later:

> When there was a large group we used to have these rounds at the beginning and end and I always used to go home feeling gauche. It's as if it links with my early proletarian upbringing . . . I haven't quite absorbed the language of the bourgeoisie – I hope it doesn't feel like the proles whinging . . . it's not that.

At another point:

> Often I feel not a full member of [group supervision] because it's on therapy issues and I obviously haven't got the same knowledge or I . . . I don't mean I feel excluded, but I don't feel such a full member.

Despite such short-comings, attempting to work cooperatively had some important pay-offs. First, all the counsellors commented on gaining a great deal of emotional support and intellectual enrichment from formal mutual supervision arrangements. These took the form of fortnightly paired two-hour sessions run on 'co-counselling' lines, where they reviewed their own cases with each other. These sessions then alternated with fortnightly group sessions addressing general issues. Given the all-round demands of their work, such arrangements seemed crucial. They also reflected the counsellors' determination to avoid falling into what they identified as the sexist psychological trap common to women: feeling it was right to wear themselves out in caring for others. This emerged as an ideal they were trying to attain, rather than the reality of day-to-day work.

> *Elspeth*: We often give up our supervision time to do other more mundane business-like things and it's not until six months later . . . we [discover] that we've given up sort of three or four of these sessions and we're wondering why we are pulling our hair out and feeling very distressed and unhappy with ourselves . . . it's because we're not giving

enough support to ourselves . . . and so we're having to struggle with that – to feel OK about giving ourselves time and making that a valid part of our work.

Second, all the counsellors and the coordinator referred to informal contact from colleagues as offering a great deal of support. Again, it reflected a view of each other as having problems in common. *Elspeth*: 'I can have a pretty difficult time and I can walk out there and I've got people out there who will hear how difficult it has been.'

Third, all the counsellors described how for them the attempt to work more cooperatively had produced the twin benefits of a creative sense of participation, and protection from being unilaterally overwhelmed by organizational demands. *Miriam*: 'It's like an increase in involvement and a decrease in responsibility – a wonderful thing – if you were running this with one person and having lots of people working under you, it would be a tremendous pressure.'

Future as an organization

During our contact the Centre was facing two problems common to feminist self-help initiatives: first, the paucity and short-term nature of funding which relatively autonomous feminist initiatives can attract; second, the danger that the relative organizational distance can make it easier for the sexism inherent in the larger institutions to go unchallenged (Rowbotham 1989: Ch. 9). The Centre's funding only had three years in total to run. No other substantial source of funding in the voluntary sector was available. Income from fees was not a solution under consideration. Therefore, on pragmatic grounds, entry into the National Health Service (NHS) had to be considered. It also held out the prospect of putting the workers in more direct contact with those already in the NHS. That feminist therapy on the NHS was an option at all was clearly due to the pioneering spadework of one counsellor, who had battled for years on committees to gain recognition for the ideals the Centre represented. At the point our contact with the Centre ceased – the workers had just heard that the local health authority had agreed to fund them on a long-term basis – their future was financially secure. Whether or not such incorporation would undermine the Centre's freedom to operate and subvert rather than preserve its aims is therefore a question for another study.

Barnes and Maple (1992) have assembled evidence indicating it is possible to make headway in promoting anti-sexist practice and policy within state mental health bureaucracies. However, both the controversial elements in such a transition and some important strategic lessons, such as the need to acquire allies within, in advance, and placement in a relatively sympathetic sector of the host organization, are highlighted in Rosemary's *cri de coeur*.

Rosemary: There was this huge fear that we were going to be kind of 'taken over' and 'mopped up' by this great bureaucratic machine . . . We've got into the Community Unit, but they're not going to come round here and tell us how to do it . . . once you get the money, you get the strings, but here was a way of getting the money without the strings . . . I want to get women's therapy into the NHS for Christ's sake, not have it 'out there'.

The pre-eminence of feminist therapy as an enterprise

The counsellors' vision of the Centre's future also revealed that organizationally they framed the solution to women's emotional distress as follows: care from a feminist perspective should be provided through individual counselling or therapeutic group work, as, or in, an agency specializing in women's emotional or mental health problems.

Rosemary: If we're going to bring about fundamental changes in psychotherapy and attitudes to women and break into traditional psychiatry and see this as a real, sort of crusade in the preventative sense, we've got to be in the establishment.

This standpoint also reflects a trend in writings on feminist therapy, e.g. Chaplin (1988), Walker (1990), Burstow (1992).

However, such a standpoint is problematic. The origins of women's emotional problems are defined as stemming from broader social conditions. Therefore, other types of feminist initiative grappling with these conditions would seem as relevant to securing women's emotional welfare as feminist therapy. For example, in relation to the physical and concomitant emotional distress of domestic violence, work on such issues as alternative housing provision and legal rights – not immediately defined as related to women's emotional wellbeing – has been shown to have important consequences for it. Moreover, such work may not comprise forms of intervention akin to feminist therapy but take the form of lobbying or advocacy (Yllö and Bograd 1988).

Nevertheless, the equal relevance of such initiatives is not acknowledged in the standpoint under discussion. Walker (1990) discusses how broader social conditions have a crucial impact on women's wellbeing, that initiatives to improve social conditions for women have profoundly affected options open to them, but still does not explore the significance of feminist initiatives other than feminist therapy for women's emotional wellbeing. The upshot is that despite aiming to work from a feminist perspective, the practitioners and commentators concerned may be trapped in the idea of feminist therapy as an enterprise being *the* appropriate organizational response to women's emotional wellbeing. As a result, their approach tends to eclipse the importance of other types of feminist initiative which may be equally relevant to women's emotional welfare.

Work in which Holland has been engaged (1989, 1990, 1992) provides an exception to this trend. Women who have participated in psychotherapy are encouraged towards activism to secure local resources conducive to their emotional wellbeing, such as resources for establishing self-help counselling. However, the main focus of such efforts remains the provision of counselling. Holland also conceptualizes emotional distress as taking forms, such as in the experience of profound loss, to which psychotherapy but not other types of activity can relate (1990). Once again this begs the question of whether intervention other than psychotherapy may not also be of relevance.

Conclusion

Evidence from the counsellors' and coordinator's accounts suggests that to some extent they developed perspectives, modes of practice and forms of organization within the Centre which addressed profound social inequalities. It also suggests that inasmuch as they were able to do so, the Centre was better able to meet the emotional needs not only of the women concerned but also the workers. However, discriminatory and elitist assumptions and practices reflective of social relations more generally, and the marginalization of women's emotional wellbeing as an issue in society at large, also eroded their egalitarian intentions. In all these respects, the indications were that experience in this location reflected more widespread tendencies in feminist therapy and also contained lessons not only for feminist therapy, but for feminist initiatives more generally.

Note 1: Gestalt therapy

Mainly developed and popularized by Fritz Perls. It concentrates on promoting emotional wellbeing with reference to people's current emotional state. It proceeds on the assumption that we all possess the emotional resources necessary for emotional wholeness or wellbeing. Through enacting by means of various exercises, what seems to be the cause of any emotional inhibition, we can come to greater awareness of what, in our own constellation of emotions, is actually blocking self-expression. One device employed is literally objectifying what seems to be hindering our efforts, e.g. by choosing a cushion or chair to represent a hostile force then directing our feelings towards it/them. In the course of doing so the aim is to express the sort of feelings that have been stirred up in us, to recognize them and their undermining effects and to lose them. For further reading on the ideas and practice informing Gestalt therapy as developed by Perls, see Perls (1969). For a useful discussion of the significance of Gestalt Therapy, particularly for work from a feminist perspective, see Ernst and Goodison (1981).

five

Like an oasis:
women's experience of
feminist therapy

Introduction

Counsellors' accounts are crucial to understanding the significance of feminist therapy. However, for a fuller understanding, women participants' views are essential. These are presented here: first, why the women in our sample sought feminist therapy; second, what they experienced as liberating about it; third, their criticisms. Finally, in addition to discussing women's own criticisms, further evidence from their accounts about limitations to feminist therapy's capacity to promote emotional wellbeing through redressing profound social inequalities is discussed. From this range of material a picture is obtained of how egalitarian are the outcomes of feminist therapy.

Why women sought feminist therapy

This emerged as being for a complex blend of reasons in which social inequalities were strongly implicated.

Substantial distress

While acknowledging that there are some women in genuine need of what feminist therapy offers, Raymond has asserted that by its existence it tends to promote 'psychological hypochondria' (1986: 156).

Contrary to Raymond's assertion, but confirming the counsellors' comments, women in our sample seemed to be seeking feminist therapy in order to resolve substantial distress. In some cases, women's emotional wellbeing had been chronically undermined. Gillian came to sort out why she could not have an orgasm – regarded as one of the most emotionally rewarding physical experiences. She saw the causes as stemming from sexual abuse as a child but had been unable to resolve them. Others faced apparently intractable dilemmas. Beatrice longed to adopt a child, but this was problematic because she had just had a mastectomy for breast cancer, and when cleared in five years time, would be judged too old. *Beatrice*: 'You're grieving for the child you never had. You don't necessarily have to have had a child and lost it to have that feeling.'

Annie's circumstances reflected how some women were beleaguered by traumatic events and caring responsibilities. She had recently had a hysterectomy following the discovery of cancer of the uterus, and was experiencing severe menopausal symptoms. Her daughter had just been diagnosed as having multiple sclerosis (MS) and had turned to Annie as her chief source of support. The medication for Annie's husband's high blood pressure had rendered him impotent, thereby undermining what had previously been a very satisfying sexual relationship for her. In addition, a major reorganization at work had taken no account of Annie's experience or interests.

Some women described acute emotional crises, *Esther*: 'I felt I was going mad. I went to my doctors and just collapsed in a sobbing heap saying I might just as well die, I couldn't live like this.' Others described quiet but mounting despair. *Jan*: 'like being up against a brick wall – wanting to be another person but feeling totally trapped in being a particular person I didn't want to be.'

Even when women described apparently moderate distress, their accounts suggested a significant degree of emotional suffering. *Katherine* initially described going to the Centre: 'post-separating from husband, post-qualifying and post-finding somewhere to live' but later commented 'I felt valueless, failed wife, failed mother, failed everything.'

The impact of social inequality

The gendered nature of women's problems was very evident. Winifred's account illustrated how the enormous expectations embedded in the caring role of wife and mother had undermined her emotional stamina.

> *Winifred*: I've always tried desperately to have a career . . . I've got an eighty-year-old mother who takes and needs a lot of support. I've got a handicapped child who needs a lot of support. I've got a criminal child, I say criminal – they say psychopath. And in the midst of this my husband is away a lot abroad, and doesn't want to get involved.

The consequences of comparative powerlessness as children also featured prominently. A few women considered their childhood experience irrelevant and the evidence supported this. Louise had specifically sought help as a result of anxieties about her subsequent health following a heart attack – a very common concern (Johnson 1991). She did not see any connection between her anxieties relating to this event and the outcome of relationships in childhood. Nor had her earlier account suggested this (Chapter 2). However, before coming to the Centre several of the women in addition to Gillian, had seen the roots of current problems as lying in childhood. *Sue* considered her compulsive eating problem as deriving partially from her situation as a child 'as a child and as an adolescent I never had anyone to talk to, someone else I could confide in.' Coming to the Centre – 'the big thing was to have someone to talk to.' Frances described how she had come to the Centre when once again the pattern of almost overwhelming anxiety at a relationship ending had repeated itself. She knew this had originated in childhood when her grandfather, who had been her one source of reliable affection had moved away.

Another group of women had sought feminist therapy for a number of apparently disparate reasons: *Zoë*: because of a spider phobia and feeling persistently miserable and lonely. *Debbie*: had felt there was 'something terribly wrong' with her as a person. *Nina*: because of the undermining effects of a very damaging relationship with another woman.

However, they all commented that as a result of interaction with the counsellors they had come to connect the way their emotional wellbeing had been undermined as children with these problems. Given the counsellors' theoretical emphasis on childhood experience as a determinant of subsequent emotional wellbeing, there is an obvious danger that women's views of the origins of their problems had been inappropriately shaped up in feminist therapy. Against this being the case, none of the women had felt mystified by their problems being redefined in this way. On the contrary, what had previously seemed to them bizarre or pathological about their own behaviour had been rendered explicable.

> *Zoë*: I was naturally sceptical about the fact that something in previous life might be making me afraid of spiders. It doesn't seem to follow through. Really my first memories of feeling this about spiders was from my early teens, just after my father died and I must have suppressed all my feelings about his death. I never admitted publicly that I was upset. I was a tough nut 'it didn't matter, nothing mattered' . . . that was the image I put out to the world, but obviously I needed some attention. And I remember in class once a spider going down the aisle and I jumped up and made a big fuss and people were sorry for me and I'd always used this to get people to help me, to get some attention . . . And almost after my first visit [to the Therapy Centre] I felt a dramatic difference in how I felt about spiders just from having talked to someone about it.

Nina spoke of the devastating impact of her relationship with a woman which had so disturbed and puzzled her that she had come to the Centre.

Nina: I more or less went expecting counselling in the short term and being very definite about the situation which was not what I got at all . . . Well, I do now but I didn't then think . . . a lot of it went back to me trying to assert myself and to convince myself I had rights, that I was a person and I think that goes back to my relationship with my mother.

Viewed independently (see Chapter 2), this group of women's accounts of their childhood relationships had also suggested that their emotional needs had been disregarded then, with profound and continuing effects on their emotional wellbeing.

Sexist and ageist aspects of social relations also featured in interaction with the impact of other social divisions in women's reasons for seeking therapy. Ruth described how chronic feelings of low self-esteem stemming from childhood had been compounded by the trauma of unemployment and the demands of coming to terms with her own lesbian identity and were the immediate precipitants of seeking feminist therapy. Louise had had the nightmarish experience of her concerns about her physical condition being dismissed by a consultant when severe chest pains had persisted after her heart attack. 'The Dr said, "Oh, you ladies."' His response represented a blend of sexism (Roberts 1985) and the disablist treatment of patients' understanding of their own physical state as of no account (Oliver 1990: Ch. 1). The net result had been to intensify Louise's anxiety, which brought her to the Centre.

The fluid nature of social hierarchies

Accounts from women in our study did not suggest that women's emotional needs were undermined because they consistently occupied a readily identifiable subordinate social position. Instead, a more fluid picture of the operation of social hierarchies and their impact on women's emotional welfare emerged. For example, Nina's account had demonstrated that another women's dominating behaviour – that of her female partner – had compounded her profound lack of self-confidence, leaving her feeling that it had virtually been destroyed. There was also evidence of women's emotional wellbeing being undermined by the consequences of the dominant social position they occupied. Winifred described herself as gaining great affection from her son with severe learning difficulties. *Winifred*: 'I know without a shadow of doubt I love my handicapped child, we're very much in tune, we can talk across a room without speech.' The heavy personal cost of caring could be seen as a major factor eroding this positive effect. But also the discriminatory tone of her previous account: 'an eighty-year-old mother', 'a handicapped child', 'a criminal child' (page 113), suggests she tended to see limits to what her mother and children could offer her because of their respective ages and cognitive and psychological states. The subordinate status she ascribed to them can thus be seen as compounding the emotional burden of caring she carried.

Christine's situation exemplified the way in which a complex sequence of shifts in power relations – in part against the trend of dominant social relations and back in line with them again – could affect women's emotional wellbeing. Christine's relationship with her male partner, which brought her to the Centre, could be seen as very much on his terms. She had been driven to distraction by the way he had disregarded her feelings. However, at the point that Christine came, the balance of power in terms of brute force was very much in her favour. Christine's anger had manifested itself in physical violence and murderous thoughts. Nevertheless, in the midst of her physical ascendancy, Christine's power was already ebbing away. This reflects the tendency of women to treat the responsibility for maintaining heterosexual relationships as their responsibility but on men's terms (Walker 1990: Ch. 1); Christine came to the Centre not to sort out her partner's behaviour as the root cause of the problem, but to curb her own behaviour – for his sake – and to do what she could to maintain their relationship.

> *Christine*: Quite frankly I was frightened of killing him . . . I know I wanted to work on the relationship and I couldn't cope with the feelings I'd got . . . That's why I went to the Centre . . . I was frightened of my own violence.

The women's accounts thereby provide a telling critique of practice as theorized by the counsellors and in current texts. Reductionist tendencies to dwell on childhood interactions and development as *the* cause of women's distress are shown to run the risk of seriously distorting its origins. Sexist social conditions both current and historical, emerge as intrinsic to the problems women bring into feminist therapy (Walker 1990). However, as Burstow (1992) has argued, social conditions representing other forms of inequality are as relevant. Moreover, women's accounts confirm that women do not consistently occupy a subordinate position, and that this too is reflected in women's emotional state. However, the evidence in women's accounts also moves on from Burstow's work, by showing that the shifting nature of the power balance in hierarchical social relations is also germane to women's emotional welfare.

The limitations of other sources of help

Women also sought feminist therapy as a result of the limitations of other potential sources of help which had left them isolated once emotional problems had arisen. Again the subordinating effects of current social relations were played out here.

Repeatedly, women had not been able to turn to those people who would be commonly designated as closest to them – husbands, partners, children, parents. This was because the nature of the relationship in question was integral to their problems! It lay at the crux of their emotional needs being undermined: see Annie's, Christine's, Frances's, Katherine's, Nina's, Ruth's, Sue's and Winifred's accounts above. Even where their 'closest' relationships did not seem to be centrally implicated in women's distress, passing comments suggested that such relationships could not be relied on as a prime source of comforting and concern. *Gillian* on her current male partner who had another sexual relationship too: 'I didn't feel comfortable with [him] 'cause he wasn't mine, I'd wake up in the morning and he'd be gone.'

In contrast to such relationships, and consistent with women's experience generally, their friendships with other women had provided some support with the problems that had brought them to the Centre. They had provided 'a listening ear' and had also acted as a channel of referral – passing on information about the Centre and encouraging women to go. *Louise*: 'Fiona saw it [i.e. the state she was in]' she said, 'why don't you go to the women's counselling thing?'

About half the women had had prior experience of other forms of professional treatment before deciding to seek feminist therapy. Five had had experience of diverse forms of counselling. The impression was that this range of counselling had had few negative effects – the strongest criticism was Irene's of bioenergetics (Ernst and Goodison 1981: 108–46) 'it was weird'. Instead counselling had been moderately helpful, but in the women's opinion had not tackled the roots of their problems.

Several women (Louise, Olivia, Zoë, Winifred, Esther and Irene) had also had medical treatment, in most cases with their GP, for the problems they brought to the Centre. This is the most common professional contact for women experiencing severe emotional problems (Barnes and Maple 1992). In a couple of cases, e.g. Louise, and Olivia, who found her consultant's response to her eating problem 'impersonal, lacking in warmth and reassurance', they had found their treatment overtly subordinating. In this way it echoed the experiences of other women, identified by advocates and theoreticians of women's therapy. But in other cases, women felt they had been treated with concern but that medical intervention had proved to be irrelevant and therefore ineffectual. For example, Winifred's doctor had given her 'some cheer up pills' then wrung his hands and commented, 'It's a tragedy; Winifred.' I said, 'I know that.' 'But they can't do anything at all.' *Irene* commented on how futile psychiatric consultations could be: 'an appointment with a psychiatrist who will sit there go "hum" and "ah" and not want to see me for another couple of months.' Women's experience therefore tended to bear out the counsellors' comments and a further tenet of feminist approaches to women's emotional health. One of the dangers of conventional medical intervention is that it can be a diversionary exercise – appearing to guarantee something is being done when it is not, and consigning women to continued suffering (Gorman 1992: 24–5).

Women as active agents

Despite the intensity of distress women felt and the lack of support they experienced, they were not simply passive victims of their emotional problems. They were actively seeking relief and to secure their wellbeing. Despite being in the depths of depression, Irene had decided to strike out from previous unsatisfactory solutions and go to the Centre.

> *Irene*: I didn't want to go off sick again and I didn't want to go on any form of medication. I had been on anti-depressants for six months and weaned myself off those 'cause my doctor said I'd be on them for a couple of years and I wasn't having that.

Despite the seemingly amorphous nature of her problems, Debbie's urge to gain relief came through. *Debbie*: 'I'd got problems but like in water and every time I'd put my hand in to fetch one out to get it out of the way, to say "that's one" and I kept thinking, "Oh I can't do this on my own, I do need some sort of help."'

The women's approach to obtaining help therefore tallied with the counsellors' concept of them as active participants in their own care, and with the feminist concept of women in the 'client' or 'patient' role as being self-determining agents (Phillips and Rakusen 1989). The wisdom of the principle of self-referral was also confirmed, as on the evidence here, women could be trusted to seek help for themselves.

The Centre's positive attractions

In the context of non-existent, limited, or inappropriate help from other sources, the Centre held positive attractions. It offered counselling free-of-charge, but above all, appealed as a women-only enterprise. Either from previous experience or general knowledge, women seemed to have a broad understanding of what counselling/therapy entailed, probably reflecting the influence of its growth. They did not seem to make a distinction between counselling or therapy (Mearns and Dryden 1990: ix–x) but defined this as an interactive relationship which concentrated on encouraging them to make sense of their problems. *Gillian*: 'I saw the Centre as a place I could sit and talk about the way I felt – not "why I didn't have an orgasm" but about my childhood and how it's affecting me now. I interpreted the title as a place to talk about problems.'

The importance of counselling being free at the Centre was commented on, several women stating that they simply could not have afforded fees for private therapy. Brown has argued that ensuring this may result, ironically, in a degree of organizational control on feminist therapists from state funding agencies, out of keeping with feminist aims (Brown 1992: 250–1). The counsellor's experience demonstrated that this is a live issue. However, it cannot be congruent with the egalitarian aims of feminist therapy for it to be available only to women above a certain minimum disposable income. Therefore the existence of funded centres is crucial.

As women spoke of what attracted them to feminist therapy, they revealed varying degrees and forms of commitment to feminist ideals. However, the nub of the Centre's attraction was its women-only nature.

Christine: Certainly because it was women only . . . I'm very unhappy about going to see a male counsellor . . . I've always turned to women to discuss and have emotional rapport with, and I just perceive the Centre, as also its feminist outlook, as being the sort of therapy that would be helping.

Mary: I didn't see it as anything apart from it was run by women for women.

Several factors seemed to coalesce to make the women-only nature of the Centre attractive: women's own tendency to turn to other women for support with what were defined as emotional problems; the experience of finding other women friends supportive; the experience of frequently finding interaction with men or male professionals unsupportive or undermining; and discrimination in respect of other social divisions. For lesbian women in the sample, the absence of an explicitly lesbian counselling centre in the area at the time and the marginalization of lesbianism in counselling and health care generally (Brown 1992), may have meant that the Centre's approach represented the most positive option available. *Tina*: 'a place for women . . . I wanted to develop and didn't know how to do it, I thought I wasn't expressing how I felt or thought to people, I wanted to be myself around people.' Women's attitude here may also have reflected a stage in the evolution of feminist ideas more generally, where the emphasis was on all-inclusive sisterhood. Hanmer and Statham, writing at the time on women and social work stated, 'Women social workers and clients share commonalities . . . These commonalities offer both a resource and a strength for practice' (1988: 9).

However, reliance on the women-only nature of the Centre as guaranteeing women's interests was problematic. It did not guarantee an appreciation of the way the operation of gender undermines women's emotional wellbeing (Walker 1990). Given that forms of inequality other than those that were gender-derived featured in women's own accounts, the focus on the guaranteed advantages of a women-only organization may have been misplaced. The attitudes of women coming into feminist therapy and those of the counsellors themselves could also compound each other, perpetuating discriminatory shortcomings in practice. For instance, none of the women in our sample specified that they required a feminist therapy centre which explicitly addressed the interests of women experiencing disability as a result of physical impairment, nor had the counsellors identified this as a requirement for their own work. Finally, if the assumption among women going to feminist therapy centres, as well as women working there, is that it is appropriate for only *women* to do the work of relieving women's emotional suffering, then this further reinforces the process of men being exonerated from responsibility for taking action to end women's distress.

Access

The counsellors worked hard at publicizing the Centre through talks, leaflets and open evenings. However, for most of the women, knowledge of the Centre came through friendship and professional networks. Typically, *Frances*: 'I knew a few women who were going to the Centre, but I can't remember whether anyone really said to me, "You ought to go to it".' Katherine had met one of the Centre's counsellors through a course connected with her work. Such word-of-mouth publicity, combined with self-referral, may have enhanced the Centre's identity as a place accessible to women. However, friendship and professional networks as the main medium for information about the Centre's existence may also have restricted access by reinforcing the predominantly white, middle-class, and comparatively youthful nature of its constituency. This point was picked up by

> *Louise*: I'm not being classist, but I wonder if it's people with higher education who get to know about it, and the people who need it more, who don't have the right education and knowledge, never hear of it. I only heard through my friend Fiona. Before marriage I worked for the NSPCC and saw a lot of poverty and cruelty and I wonder if these sort of women get to know about it.

Women's accounts of why they came to the Centre reflected the interplay of various dimensions to inequality, but were also marked by the absence of certain dimensions, reflecting the exclusive nature of the Centre's constituency. For example, although the undermining effects of living in long-term poverty have been heavily implicated in women's emotional distress (Payne 1991: Ch. 6), these did not feature. Nor, for example, did the undermining effects of the interaction of gender, poverty and racism (Commission for Racial Equality 1993). Certain populations of women were also absent – women with learning difficulties and much older women. The consequences were that the requirements of the same populations of women which feminist practice more generally has been identified as tending to marginalize seemed also marginalized in feminist therapy (Langan and Day 1992). Second, the importance of initiatives to reach women in such circumstances, through work on the location, organization and philosophy of feminist therapy and counselling is underlined (Holland 1989; Laws 1991). Finally, it suggests that any benefits gained from feminist therapy as represented in the experience of this sample, should be seen to accrue to a group of women in selected social circumstances.

Women's experience of feminist therapy: introduction

Women came into feminist therapy as a selected population in a state of substantial distress, in which the effects of social inequalities were heavily implicated. They had not obtained relief elsewhere, but considered that the chance of non-hierarchical counselling with other women would enable them to achieve this.

Their accounts demonstrated that in feminist therapy, in contrast to other relationships, nearly all the women most of the time had the following comparatively rare experience of freedom from subordination. Their emotional needs were treated as important and their capacity to contribute to their own and others' emotional wellbeing was valued. As a result of this opportunity to be their truer (i.e. less subordinated) selves in these respects, women experienced a greater sense of self-worth and consequently felt happier. This state of comparative wellbeing also seemed to endure, despite otherwise inclement social conditions. By promoting women's emotional wellbeing in this way, feminist therapy could be seen as contributing to creating more egalitarian social relations.

This positive outcome is analysed first, before the limitations to feminist therapy – also suggested by the women's accounts – are discussed. A variety of processes seemed to produce the effect of women's emotional needs and capabilities *not* being subordinated. These are set out in turn, but as this is done, their interlocking nature becomes apparent.

The positive nature of women's experience

Freedom of expression

Women's desire to express what troubled them had an outlet. It was not thwarted as had frequently been the case in previous relationships in childhood and adulthood, including those involving various practitioners. *Annie*: 'Ventilation. It was like opening the floodgates – everything poured out at once.' *Louise*: 'It did me a world of good to pour all this out, because I couldn't tell my doctor . . . talking over my head as if I was a little animal.' *Irene* described a similar phenomenon in the group she'd been in at the Centre 'an atmosphere . . . where I could start talking about things I'd never really talked about before'.

Women didn't refer to the confidentiality of the relationship with the counsellor or in the groups as crucial to being able to express what was important to them, but to other facets of the relationship, discussed next, both significant in their own right and in conjunction with each other.

Emotional needs and capabilities not treated as inferior

Over and over again, women described how the unusual experience of not having their feelings and efforts defined as inferior began to make them feel better. *Frances*: 'complete acceptance that I could be and do anything and it was OK and that was what was really important'. *Debbie*: 'a very special relationship where I could say how I really felt without any come-back or withdrawal or resentment'. *Irene* on the group she was in: 'I feel anything I do and say there can be accepted – I still don't feel I've got that sort of confidence in other relationships, so I'm much more cagey. I feel the closest I can be to myself is in the group.' *Winifred*: 'What helped me tremendously is her saying, "There is a reason for this and it's not your fault."' Only rarely had this been a feature of previous relationships in childhood or in adulthood and then for the most part with women friends.

However, women also commented on how, unlike in their friendships, there was no threat of losing face. In this way they revealed how important it had been to maintain equivalence of status in friendship and not risk the slide into a subordinate role.

> *Christine*: Initially relief at having someone to talk to who wasn't involved in my life . . . to be able to talk without having to colour it, because I think you tend to colour your perceptions of what the problems are depending on the friend.

The opportunity to concentrate on their own emotional needs

In another way the relationship with the counsellors transcended that offered by the best of friends. Women were freed from the responsibility of caring for someone else's emotional wellbeing at the same time as their own. The risk that their interests would take second place was thereby further reduced. That caring for the other party's wellbeing had been routine in other relationships was revealed by women's comments on how unusual the situation with the counsellor felt. *Nina*: 'The one thing that struck me about it was it was very one-sided and I think that I never got over the oddness of that.' Odd or not, such an arrangement had a conspicuous impact on enabling women to register the importance of their own needs.

> *Katherine*: She made that quite clear at the beginning. She was there for me and I mustn't look after her . . . I couldn't get used to that at first . . . but she was quite strict about it . . . And in the end I got used to that – because for an hour a week it was just me and what I wanted to talk about . . . I've never really had that before, nobody every invested that much in me without there being some sort of price to pay, without sounding too cynical . . . I used to love it . . . You get really hungry for it.

Contrary to what the counsellors had feared, participating in group work at the centre, as opposed to one-to-one counselling, did not rule out the possibility of a similar effect. It seemed to come about through women identifying problems in common. As other women in the group discussed *their* problems, so the discussion could be as relevant to the individual who was listening as if her own problems were being discussed.

> *Irene*: And listening to women discussing the problems they were having . . . There were a lot of things said I could identify with, it made me more ready to accept on a conscious level feelings I'd got about my mother, whereas I'd felt like a lot of women that it wasn't acceptable for a daughter to hate her mother.

Tina: 'It was quite amazing – the shared experience – though we had differing experiences, we could still relate to each other.' This corroborates existing findings identifying such a process as a strength of feminist group work (Donnelly 1986; Butler and Wintram 1991: Ch. 4).

Being cared for

As distinct from much previous experience in childhood and adulthood, women also described how they felt that the counsellors and coordinator had genuinely cared about their welfare. This had boosted their sense of self-worth and had encouraged them to express themselves. *Debbie* on her counsellor: 'Caring, she actually listened. She cared how far along the path I'd gone or what I'd experienced. I think the care – between love and care – I felt it was caring.' Olivia had only had one assessment interview at the Centre but echoed the same theme –

> *Olivia*: I was made to feel I had a right to be there . . . I think there are very few people I've known in my life who've listened and let me say

what I think and that was OK. Whether they agreed or not . . . although it was only a short time, they were genuinely concerned. It wasn't just a one way thing . . . just me speaking my mind, there was some feedback.

Tina: feeling there was somewhere you could go and talk and be accepted . . . it hasn't been there in other places. At the Centre there was a genuine desire to help people.

Although *Gillian* was to voice criticisms of what she gained from the Centre, she too commented on the warm ambience, 'They were all friendly – in reception, very nice. I did feel tense at first but they made you feel comfortable as you walked in.'

Encouragement to confront and revise negative frames of reference

Women identified a further dimension to interaction with the counsellors which had boosted their self-esteem. They had been encouraged to confront and revise the negative frames of reference which others and they themselves had applied to their feelings and actions. As women's earlier accounts had indicated, these frames of reference could represent deep-seated feelings and beliefs, instilled as a result of powerful influences, or interaction with others in positions of power in their lives. Confrontation took two forms: first, being offered alternative, more positive interpretations, and second, being encouraged to confront negative frames of reference and to work out and adopt more positive views.

Beatrice: I wish I could remember now the questions she put to me but certainly I know that she reassured me that I was normal . . . I was thinking are these true feelings about adoption, about having a baby . . . I didn't feel ashamed of how I felt, just mixed up.

Sue: After I'd talked to the lady – she helped me see enough I think . . . And she told me then, people get into marriages, think it's going to be alright – they have reservations but they still do it, and perhaps I'd been quite brave to soldier on, really.

Winifred: I was assured that it wasn't wrong to have aspirations of your own. Because I really had, I do feel, lost a lot of my life.

Women themselves were also encouraged to face and reconsider their own ingrained habits and attitudes which may have undermined their emotional wellbeing. They described the counsellors – as not carrying out the labour themselves, but supporting them as they did so. This approach averted the danger of reinforcing the pathologizing idea that the women were incapable of directing their own energies towards their own wellbeing. At the same time women had the chance to exercise their capacity for self-expression –

commented on in previous chapters and in the discussion of the spirit in which they sought feminist therapy.

Katherine: She gave me the ability to identify my needs. She did that in quite a traumatic way. What she said was, 'I want you to write down what you identify as your needs' and I couldn't write down bloody anything because I didn't know. So she made me think in those areas. How could I ever get my needs met if I didn't even know what they were?

Jan: I think that was the largest part really, her making me express feeling in front of her and her saying it was perfectly alright for me to do this, 'I'm not going to be washed away by your tears, people do cry – it's not anything' . . . I was actually able to say to her I resented her for doing that . . . and I spent a lot of time telling her I found it really difficult to express anger or to have arguments with people . . . that you could feel angry with someone and have a huge row with them and they could still love you . . . I think most of my memory was that if there was an argument of any sort I would end a relationship.

Length of time in feminist therapy

Finally, nearly all the women commented on how they felt that the length of time in feminist therapy devoted to their emotional needs had been appropriate. Again this contrasted with their experience in other relationships and forms of treatment. The counsellors had emphasized that their policy was to offer women they could take on, non-time-limited counselling, to counter what they saw as the tendency to minimize the attention paid to women's emotional needs.

On the evidence here, with three qualifications, the counsellors' concern had paid off. First, Gillian felt that one-and-a-half hour sessions would have provided nearer the time she needed to express her feelings. None of the other women commented on finding the requirement of hourly sessions constraining. Some also described feeling quite tired by the end of them. The second major qualification arose from the constraints posed by the Centre's shortage of resources. This was not the responsibility of the counsellors, but it meant that most women who contacted the Centre for counselling did not end up having any time in feminist therapy. The further test of the negative effects of the shortage of resources was the position of women having one-off assessment interviews once the waiting list was closed. Did women express a need for longer contact which was simply closed off to them? All the women in this position in our sample commented on how just one interview had boosted their self-esteem and happiness in an enduring way. However, Olivia had felt the need for more time.

Olivia: The only thing is I wish I had a lasting contact, because it's a very valuable support system, and I could benefit from it, I'm sure other women could if they had the resources . . . I think I still need some kind of contact and support.

Otherwise, only *Jan* commented that she 'would have liked to carry on longer'. For the rest of the women, with lengths of contact varying between three months and three years (see Appendix 2), the time had seemed to be appropriate, neither too short nor too long. The work of sorting this out seemed to be characterized by fine tuning on their part and the counsellors', with the women's interests uppermost. *Esther*, on the circumstances in which she finally decided to stop going to the Centre, 'She was very reassuring, I felt they weren't going to cut me off till I wanted . . . and when I did want . . . it was good, I felt OK.' *Debbie*: 'I'd gone along the road as far as I could in rapid change, and I felt I would have been wasting time if I continued . . . No more could be done via counselling, it was up to me to go along the path I started out on.' On the pragmatic grounds of servicing a wider population, time-limited counselling or therapy may be appropriate (Kareem and Littlewood 1992). However, the evidence from these women's experience is that while long-running contact may not be necessary for women's needs to be met, having the length of contact appropriate to their needs is important, if they are to benefit from counselling or therapy.

The results of women's positive experience of feminist therapy

The results of women having an experience of relative freedom from their emotional needs and emotional resources being treated as inferior, were striking. From feeling 'failures', 'mad' or 'overwhelmed', they began to feel a sense of self-worth and consequently happiness. It was as though they had come into the sunshine.

Debbie: 'She cared, she nurtured me, identified that I needed to give myself time, space and confidence, here's the way to build it . . . I feel like a new person.' *Louise*: 'She lifted a great load off me, and because of that contact I was better off for it . . . she made me feel a lot better. I was able to face life in general more fully than before I saw her.' *Nina*: 'It was basically getting to like myself and accept what I had been given . . . a terribly fundamental shift in attitude.'

Jan: I started to feel a lot more self-accepting, I wasn't this terrible person I'd been making myself out to be . . . I started to feel less desperate, things were returning to normal again. Probably the biggest thing about going to the Centre is me acknowledging I've got a right to be happy, as happy as possible now, rather than postponing my right to happiness.

For Frances the effects reached into her physical state.

Frances: I started to feel real . . . it put a different perspective on the rest of my life, it was just incredible. My energy level was just completely different because the things I started to deal with were the real things going on around me, rather than the things I was carrying inside me all the time.

Tina's initial session of counselling had left her feeling 'high and wonderful, I went out and bought a bunch of flowers, it was like having my thoughts arranged . . . instead of in a jumble'.

This change in women's emotional state represents a massive achievement, set against the scale of their previous distress and the input of previous relationships and treatment. Years in what would have been defined as close relationships and well established state-funded treatment had not eased, but for the most part compounded the acute and chronic distress which women had suffered. Yet engagement in feminist therapy had lifted this.

The predisposing factors enabling this to come about seemed to be: the women's own approach; the counsellors' and coordinator's commitment and hard work; the application of some of the main planks of the counsellors' theories; the organization of the Centre and the fruits of more widespread feminist activism. These are discussed next.

Predisposing factors in meeting women's emotional needs and requirements

Women's active engagement

Women did not fall into the passive patient mode once they began feminist therapy. Their determination to secure a better emotional state for themselves continued. The evidence from their accounts was that, with the right conditions, they could begin to experience a greater degree of emotional wellbeing, and that they shared with the counsellors in creating these conditions. Evidence of women's input also endorsed the counsellors' impression that they displayed considerable psychological fortitude as they confronted what could be quite deep-seated feelings and beliefs.

Tina, on going to her group: 'I always hated going, but it's like if you go and speak you might reveal things, emotions, but on the other side I wanted to do it, it's like being afraid but knowing it will do you good.'

Debbie: [My counsellor] identified the rejection I felt from my Mum – and the rejection I felt from my first husband. Then when I met my second husband I was so overwhelmed by the love I couldn't believe, I could not come to terms with it. She identified I said to her, 'I'm going to cry if you ask me about love.' It's strange I don't cry when I talk about rejection. I never ever realized it before. I never linked it in with anything except that I was perhaps over the top. She identified that to me, and I thought, 'Why didn't I think that?' You experience it too many times.

The counsellors' commitment and hard work

The depth of the counsellors' personal commitment to women's right to secure their emotional wellbeing has come through in women's preceding accounts. However, descriptions of the counsellors' input also highlighted their concentration and attention to detail.

> *Christine*: The most powerful session was where we went back and did a memory lifescript, message from mother, grandmother, grandfather, where they'd led to, what feelings they'd led to. . . And that was really powerful and extremely useful. I've kept it, to look at when I want it.

None of the women at any point in the interviews mentioned counsellors being unpunctual, or forgetting an appointment, or cancelling without warning. Any of these things could have undermined women's feelings that the counsellors cared about them.

The application of a range of theories

The counsellors' feminist perspective could be seen as enabling them to appreciate the tendency for women and other parties to treat women's behaviour and feelings as inferior, and to challenge this. Otherwise feminist tenets seemed to coalesce with those from counselling and psychotherapy in various ways to positive effect, as, for example, in the way the counsellors regarded women as active agents in tackling the emotional problems they faced. (See Nelson-Jones 1988: Ch. 1; Woodward 1988: Ch. 8 for further discussion in relation to counselling and psychotherapy respectively.) Again, a central principle of the practice of counselling and psychotherapy, also implicit in a feminist approach, was the way counsellors had made it clear that they would not pass judgement on women's attitudes and behaviour (see Oldfield 1983: Ch. 2). The origins of instituting open-ended time scales for contact may have lain in psychotherapy but were reinforced by the determination to give women a fairer deal. In the same way, feminist, psychotherapeutic and some counselling (but not co-counselling) practice converged to establish the ground rule that within feminist therapy women should be freed from caring about meeting the emotional needs of the counsellor. This did not mean that the counsellor stood aloof, but that the prime focus of the interaction was the women's needs (see Jacobs 1984 and Thorne 1984 respectively for further discussion of this aspect of psychotherapy and person-centred counselling). Psychotherapeutic and feminist perspectives were present in the importance attached to 'revisiting the scene of the crime' in childhood, i.e. recalling and confronting the interactions with adults which had led to distressing inhibitions being acquired then (Ernst and Goodison 1981: Ch. 8).

Offering interpretations or challenges to clients' current viewpoints may form one element in counselling and psychotherapy (Egan 1975). The women's accounts suggested that where counsellors' interpretations were informed by a feminist concern about women not individually or collectively pathologizing themselves, this was found to be helpful. The emphasis on greater assertiveness can be seen as deriving both from feminist and counselling axioms (Ernst and Goodison 1981: Ch. 1). A blend of feminist consciousness-raising and group work theory was discernible in the focus on identifying the common, gendered nature of problems which women had experienced in groupwork at the Centre (Butler and Wintram 1991).

The Centre's organization

Women's comments also reflected the importance of the ambience created in any feminist therapy centres. Women's self-esteem had clearly benefited from attempts to make the Centre's organization friendly and informal. This had enabled them to feel more relaxed and confident and therefore in a better position to benefit from counselling. The counsellors' high level of concentration, in interaction with the women, the strong sense that the counsellors' needs for support were met outside the sessions, and the clarity of feedback they gave all suggested that the emphasis on well thought out administrative routines, collective support and supervision brings dividends.

The fruits of feminist activism

Such a positive outcome can also be linked to a more general shift in power relations in society. There was no discernible difference in women's own social position before and after feminist therapy. Nevertheless, women can be seen as benefiting from the following shift in prevailing power relations: the mass of contemporary feminist activism designed to secure an equitable existence for women. One consequence of this activism had been the development of feminist therapy, as at the Centre. Women's experience there demonstrated that feminist therapy provided to some extent a bulwark against existing hierarchical social relations and a clearing in which less subordinating relations had a chance to exist.

The enduring effects of feminist therapy

Women were interviewed six months or longer after feminist therapy had finished, but it was clear that its positive effects endured. *Annie*: 'I felt restored to myself. And so I was able to go forward with much more energy – no it hasn't worn off, it's lasted. You see me restored, as far as I'm going to be.'

> *Jan*: I don't ever feel as totally despairing as I did at the point when I went to the Centre. I couldn't ever remember feeling really happy . . . feeling I was getting what I wanted emotionally. At all. Whereas now I actually feel I'm getting a lot more of what I want.

> *Christine*: I think I found [my counsellors'] evaluation of what life was like for me – and she did it very clearly . . . helpful during the period when I was looking at my relationship . . . That's something . . . I want to carry forward with me. And something that still stays with me . . . two years on.

For Nina the effect of therapy had increased since finishing 'got stronger . . . I don't think I've ever felt so good in all my life. It's coloured everything, its the result of the sessions.' *Beatrice* felt she had benefited long term but no longer consciously thought about it: 'I'm better. I don't think about it.'

The persistence of the effects of therapy didn't depend on frequent 'topping up' contacts with the Centre. Several women commented on the option of such a contact as being reassuring, but only Winifred had taken advantage of it. Given the multiple demands she faced, this seemed a reasonable provision and she was quite clear-sighted about its purpose. *Winifred*: 'If I feel a bit desperate . . . it lets off steam to a certain extent . . . I don't think she can tell me anything new to be honest.' Otherwise, several women commented on how drawing on a model of the interaction they had had in feminist therapy, in their mind's eye, had been sustaining. *Esther*: 'When I go through bad times, I use the therapy session, go back to things that occur there and tell myself things the therapist told me, I use the strength they gave me without the physical bodies . . . so the effect is still there.'

Women's more positive approach also did not seem to emanate from some facile view that they 'held the secret of life' and that from now on it would become easier. On the contrary there was ample evidence from their accounts that in various ways life had not become easier and that they were aware of this. Relationships that were important to them had ended. Katherine had started another relationship which didn't work out.

> *Katherine*: It was ever so painful. It was another rejection . . . I dealt with it, and recovered from it, it took a long time, but I think what I

learned through counselling was the ability to deal with it, rationalize it, not to take it on board as my fault, or undervalue myself . . . I didn't do that.

Current partnerships were still fraught. *Annie* spoke of continuing problems with 'My marital relationship, because we still haven't sorted it, and it looks as if it's still drifting, doing nothing.' *Christine* spoke of 'failure to establish an emotional rapport . . . the relationship is on a very difficult footing'.

Women also recognized that there were sides to their own characters that were still going to make life painful for them. Esther, had been trying to face up to living on her own for the first time in her life. However, she also commented,

> *Esther*: I suppose they [emotional problems] are different, phasing into reality rather than wanting the dream world. But they're similar. I have my insecurities, fears and worries . . . having awareness of yourself can be quite annoying, you can see well – 'come on, it's you doing this that or the other, so stop it'.

One of the spin-offs from feminist therapy which women did point to as making life easier was greater assertiveness on their own part. Sue described coming under heavy pressure at work to accept a transfer that would have amounted to a serious deterioration in working conditions. However, she thought the confidence she had gained from contact with the Centre had enabled her to resist it, because she now felt 'You musn't let people walk on you, you're important.' In terms of her personal life *Irene* commented: 'I used to feel "I can't tell people this, that or the other about myself because it's unacceptable", but now I feel it's part of me, important, and if people want to know me they'll have to hear it. If they don't like it that's their problem.'

In sum, for nearly all the women in the sample, the experience of feminist therapy emerged as being of immense and continuing benefit. *Debbie*'s comment epitomized this: 'counselling did a wonderful thing really for my life . . . I feel a general feeling of wellbeing.'

Women's criticisms of feminist therapy

Introduction

Women's criticisms were few. However, they confirmed that positive outcomes from feminist therapy only occurred when women's emotional needs and capabilities were *not* subordinated. When subordinating forms of interaction occurred, benefits to women's emotional wellbeing did not result.

The limiting effects of counsellors as 'authorities'

There was evidence that the relationship between counsellors and the women could take the form of the counsellor being an authority on practice relating to women's emotional well-being, who could not be confronted. When this happened, although the women privately realized that their emotional needs were not being met, they felt they could not challenge what was going on – to their loss.

The most poignant case concerned Gillian, the one woman in the sample who had major reservations about feminist therapy. She commented that it had provided time to think, and had resulted in her being determined to find more time for self-expression amongst the claims of her daily routine. However, she also commented 'I was glad I didn't have to go any more.' She then described how she had not found the counsellor's response supportive, but on the contrary undermining.

> *Gillian*: I saw it from her point of view as well as my own. Like I was talking about the right things. I did try to make myself talk about the problem and let her help me with it, but being uncomfortable. I told her the bits she wants to know to help me.

But while making these efforts, besides feeling uncomfortable, Gillian had also felt she was boring the counsellor, so had lied about feeling better, to bring counselling to an end. Describing her difficulty in finding someone she could express love to, since she had finished going to the Centre, Gillian sounded as alone as ever. *Gillian*: 'It's just a scaredy feeling, to know you can love, but are scared to love' . . . 'I avoid going out for one. Avoid looking at somebody if they're looking at me. Avoid them.'

Although less searing, Mary's experience was along similar lines. She had originally felt unable to challenge the counsellor's way of working which had left her mystified.

> *Mary*: The criticism I would make and I've learned since it's how you work in that sort of counselling/therapy – I was expecting someone to say, 'OK, this is what you do.' And I used to think, 'Oh my God, what am I getting from this?' She ums and ahs, repeats what I say, never gives an opinion. And that's what I needed.

Esther had found that the counsellor's favoured theoretical slant had distorted her experience during substantial tracts of counselling – 'Well the thing about my childhood was . . . let's see . . . it was irrelevant. I wanted to talk about now, it was the future I was so desperate about not my past . . . honestly I had a happy childhood so I didn't think it would help.'

Organizational shortcomings

Women's criticisms here echoed the theme that for them to benefit from the Centre, their interests needed to be met, not subordinated. The suggestion was made that women users should have greater representation in management, highlighting a shortcoming pinpointed in earlier discussion of the counsellors' approach and the organization of other feminist therapy initiatives (see Chapter 4). *Irene* on her groups' experience: 'But who is this Centre for? Is it for women who use it for their groups? And if it is shouldn't we have representatives from the groups on the management committee . . . To my knowledge this hasn't ever been asked.' Institutionalizing women's choice of counsellor was also suggested.

> *Frances*: You go the first time and you get interviewed by somebody to find out if it's mutually agreeable, I wonder how many women if they don't get a counsellor they feel they can work with, are able to say, 'Can I see somebody else?'

Gillian's situation discussed earlier illustrates the importance of this.

Marginalizing women's differential experience

Women's criticisms also suggested that their emotional needs were subordinated by their differential experience as Black women, lesbian women, women from working-class backgrounds and older women being marginalized in various ways in practice at the Centre. Thus their experience indicated that feminist therapy cannot be assumed to take account of women's differential experience in practice.

The importance of staff at the Centre having direct experience of different aspects of inequality if they were to respond adequately to women's needs was raised by Jan. She suggested that without shared experience, aspects of women's suffering could be neglected through lack of awareness. She described herself as gaining a great deal from contact with her counsellor and commented that despite her counsellor not being lesbian herself, there were issues relating to Jan's lesbian relationships she had helped with. However, Jan also described how counselling, uninformed by first-hand experience of her own sexual and class identity, had resulted in major difficulties being unaddressed. *Jan*: 'There were particular pains associated with lesbian relationships where it would have been useful to have felt I was talking to someone who had a common understanding.' There were also aspects to her feelings of lack of self-worth which she felt derived from her working-class background and might be commonplace, but again she felt that these went beyond the agenda the counsellor was prepared to tackle:

> *Jan*: I would avoid mentioning a lot of the things I felt, like anger about the class issue because I didn't want to make her uncomfortable. She was quite clear her experience was as a middle-class woman. I was terribly careful about what I said. I think [my counsellor] was very aware. When she stopped counselling she said 'I think you've said as much as you're going to say to me.'

The issue of counsellors and participants sharing direct experience of inequality remains controversial in feminist therapy. Burstow argues that it is possible for counsellors to respond in a way that is useful, through awareness and sensitivity to what such conditions may be, even if they lack first-hand experience of them (Burstow 1992: Ch. 5). Another school of thought in feminist therapy and counselling endorses Jan's standpoint and is in favour of staffing policies following suit (Laws 1991). There are two problems with this approach. First, there is no guarantee that women counsellors sharing first-hand experience may necessarily be alert to the need to challenge associated inequalities. By extension there is also no guarantee that simply setting up a 'self-help group' will be the answer. Second, as understanding of the highly differentiated nature of women's experience develops (Hughes and Mtezuka 1992), it may be difficult for staffing policies to reflect this very precisely.

However, there is evidence in writings from lesbian women (Perkins 1991) and black women (Shah 1989) that it is only as women organize on the basis of what is shared experience of social divisions other than gender, that its significance for shaping the emotional wellbeing of the women themselves starts coming out. Moreover, evidence is beginning to come through that women's experience of counselling benefits from this process. For example, an account of South Asian women's experience of emotional distress and counselling demonstrates that the South Asian women who were experiencing emotional distress recognized that women counsellors and participants at a South Asian Drop-in Centre were likely to have some understanding of the daunting circumstances they were up against, based on their own experience. Therefore, the women concerned felt able to give a fuller account of what their actual worries were. 'I go to the Asian Drop-In Centre at the Inner City Mental Health Project [ICMHP]. There I can talk to the workers and the other women who come there. It's very good for me' (Commission for Racial Equality 1993). In this way they were able to break out of the trap that Jan, in our study, had found herself in.

Corroborative evidence of the importance of access to such support comes from Gillian's experience. As an African-Caribbean woman, the lack of engagement Gillian experienced with her counsellor may not have been grounded in the limitations to the counsellor's experience as a white woman. However, given the preceding evidence, the option of an African-Caribbean woman counsellor or self-help group – neither of which were available at the Centre at the time – might have provided the opportunity for greater rapport and solidarity. The significance of this not being available is underlined by the fact that the importance of Gillian's experience as an African-Caribbean woman did not surface as an issue at any point in her account of counselling.

Women's accounts also illustrated how women's differential experience was not only marginalized in interactions between counsellors and women at the Centre. It occurred in interactions between women themselves. In Tina's account of her group she described how 'we got on well with each other, apart from one who dropped out. She was older and found it a bit intimidating.' Women also displayed discriminatory attitudes towards themselves in respect of their own differential experience as women. This was exemplified in Anne's ageist view of her self-identity in commenting that a shortfall in the Centre's provisions was a group for 'menopausal women' needed for moral support, because 'we're all disintegrating'.

In fact, movement on the issue of women's differential experience is relative to the state of women participants' own consciousness as well as that of counsellors. For example, in our sample, only one woman – Jan – already active in lesbian consciousness-raising groups, raised the importance of this as an issue.

Critique of existing inequalities being replicated in funding

Otherwise, women's criticisms did not focus on the Centre, but on the sexist nature of society for failing to meet women's need for relief from distress once it had arisen. Women identified the poor material conditions of the Centre as one consequence of this. *Christine*: 'Physically the location was not very pleasant. The rooms are very small, you could sometimes hear people crying through the walls, which was off-putting.' *Debbie*: 'There was a chap used to live upstairs and get drunk and bang about, shouting and bawling, effing and blinding, and that was a bit off-putting at times. When we got to a sensitive subject, I was listening to him.'

Above all, women attributed the lack of financial resources for the sort of work the Centre carried out to callous disregard of women's emotional welfare. In doing so they both demonstrated feelings of solidarity with other women, and once again how grateful they were for what they had gained from feminist therapy.

> *Katherine*: I am a very strong advocate of the Centre, I get angry because there should be more facilities, more resources, more of that

type of unit. I don't know what the take-up is but I imagine it's been overwhelming . . . I think, 'You bastards can't you see . . . we need this.' Not just a class of women, it's women *per se*, whatever walk of life, *women* have problems related to them as women.

Christine: I've tried to refer lots of women here but of course they've closed their waiting lists a long time ago . . . there are women out there absolutely desperate for self-validation and some healing, and I certainly got that at the Centre.'

Feminist therapy's positive outcomes therefore led to a pool of support amongst women participants for counselling initiatives to promote women's emotional wellbeing. Women emerging with a positive experience from feminist therapy could therefore be seen as politicized to the extent of being committed to the development of initiatives to meet women's need for relief from emotional distress, once it had arisen. However, they did not adopt the more radical approach of arguing that efforts should be concentrated on ending the conditions that gave rise to women's distress in the first place.

Further limitations to egalitarian outcomes

Introduction

Despite the benefits women had experienced in feminist therapy, their accounts had also suggested that there was no *guarantee* that feminist therapy provided an experience of comparative freedom from women's emotional needs and resources being treated as inferior. Their descriptions of their social circumstances as they sought feminist therapy and their experience within it indicated that when they felt that their or other women's emotional needs and resources were subordinated, this was largely due to two things: the counsellors' role amounting to professional elitism and women's differential experience of social conditions tending to be marginalized in its practice.

In addition to direct criticism, women's accounts provided evidence of further limitations to the egalitarian nature of feminist therapy's outcomes: first, the capacity for dominating behaviour by other parties in women's lives tended not to be engaged with; second, women's capacity for dominating behaviour tended not to be addressed; third, women's attention was deflected from the need for more widespread social change to promote emotional wellbeing. Finally, women's accounts indicated that even when their emotional wellbeing improved through feminist therapy, initiatives beyond it were necessary to tackle the unequal social conditions which obstructed even greater wellbeing.

Other party's dominating behaviour

Women's accounts confirmed that as a focal point of practice, counsellors did not encourage women to challenge other party's dominating behaviour, nor did they do so themselves. The two exceptions were Annie's case where the counsellor had contacted the consultant treating her and arranged a further appointment for Annie to tackle him about distressing and unwarranted side effects of treatment. In Christine's case the counsellor visited Christine's partner to help defuse the inflammatory situation by obtaining his view of things and to encourage him to consider the effects of his actions. Otherwise the focus in both one-to-one and group work remained firmly on the women concentrating on themselves to repair the emotional damage they had sustained. Winifred's experience exemplifies this approach.

> *Winifred*: She [the counsellor] has helped me come to terms with my husband and his non-accountability . . . a lot. And she's made me realize he's not being bloody-minded, it's just the way he is, the conditions of his childhood have made him non-accountable, whereas mine have made me accountable . . . so she's made me feel more sympathetic and she's made me feel not so guilty about wanting something for myself, which is hard.

The counsellors' practice here not only reflects a general tendency in one-to-one therapeutic counselling and therapeutic group work, but also feminist practice in these areas (Walker 1990 and Butler and Wintram 1991). It can be argued that another individual's behaviour may not necessarily be implicated in the emotional problems someone is experiencing. Alternatively, until women feel strong enough in themselves, it may be difficult for them to assert their own interests (Walker 1990: Ch. 8). However, there are several dangers to this approach. First, counselling or therapy may then serve to exonerate other people of the responsibility to rectify a damaging situation. Second, it may obscure the need for alternative forms of intervention to deal with the causes of women's distress. Third, it may be stigmatizing to women by implying that the roots of the problem lie in their attitude. These dangers are present in Winifred's account in microcosm. Her husband comes under no pressure to change his behaviour, and strategies to promote such a change are not considered. Meanwhile Winifred's own attitude becomes the sole target for change.

Arguing that opening up interactive strategies lies beyond the bounds of counselling practice is also no real defence. Even if the possible strategies are restricted to those readily emanating from counselling, various options open up. Remaining with men's dominating behaviour as the case in point. Counsellors could become involved in encouraging, initiating or collaborating in the development of groups for men, addressing the emotional consequences of men's sexist behaviour. Alternatively, for women's male partners, they could provide information about or encouragement towards men's one-to-one work, or men's groups tackling these issues. In doing so, counsellors would be undertaking a type of practice which still tends to be seen as on the margins of feminist action. However, examples exist and they represent a more equitable division of labour in the creation of a more egalitarian experience of emotional wellbeing. For instance, there is evidence that the importance of men taking the initiative in addressing the issue of the consequences of their behaviour for women's behaviour has become a focus of men's anti-sexist groups (Metcalf and Humphries 1985).

Women's capacity for dominating behaviour

There was also no evidence that women's capacity to behave in a dominating way was generally identified and tackled as an issue in feminist therapy. We know from the women's own accounts that their own behaviour could be dominating and that women more generally, for example in the role of parents and partners, could behave oppressively. If feminist therapy avoids this as an issue, it cannot contribute to challenging such behaviour.

The negative side to the fusion of one of the traditions of psychoanalytic and counselling practice and a facet of feminism is evident here. In psychotherapy and counselling, the counsellor adopting a non-judgemental standpoint toward the participants' accounts has been seen as essential to enabling them to divulge and review to the fullest extent the nature of problems as they see them (Oldfield 1983). One by-product of feminism has been a tendency to treat women as victims of violence and oppression and not as its perpetrators (Langan and Day 1992). The exposure of the scale on which women have been the objects of physical violence, sexual violence, financial exploitation and intellectual dominance has acted as a powerful reinforcement of this idea.

From the women's accounts, the exception to the rule of not challenging women's dominating behaviour provides a possible model for how this issue may be grappled with in feminist therapy. Both Christine and her counsellor thought there was a real danger of Christine killing her partner. As Christine's self-esteem had been increasingly undermined by her partner's disregard of her feelings, so she had come to respond with violence. Paradoxically, the counsellor's compassionate response to the violence and guilt Christine felt broke the vicious circle that had led to the violence: *Christine*: 'her non-judgemental attitude that it's OK to have jealousy, anger, violence . . . all the things that society dictates is not on . . . influenced my own self-opinion, it was at an all time low . . . she built me up and sent me out.' However, at the same time, the counsellor had challenged Christine's attitudes and behaviour which threatened another person's wellbeing. She had encouraged Christine to re-examine some of her own frames of reference towards men, including the low valuation on all male human life that Christine's grandmother had dinned into her, 'All men are bastards, Christine.' The counsellor had also drawn the line on violence. At the start of therapy she had asked Christine to give an undertaking 'a simple verbal contract' that she would not kill her partner.

Adopting the approach of retaining compassion for women behaving oppressively, tempered by challenging their oppressive behaviour, is in line with an emerging tendency in feminist work. For example, in feminist research and practice it is being acknowledged that, although apparently in a minority of instances, women do act as perpetrators of sexual abuse towards children. This may be understood in terms of the influence of dominant ideology which legitimates the treatment of people as sexual objects and the power over children that adults have. Nevertheless the oppressive effects of women's behaviour is being logged and addressed in practice with women (Elliott 1993).

Deflecting attention from the need for more widespread social change

Women's accounts confirmed the following impression from the counsellors' accounts. In feminist therapy they were not encouraged to consider the need for initiatives beyond therapy or to challenge and change widespread social conditions implicated in undermining their emotional wellbeing. Instead, their attention and energies were focused on individual solutions through feminist therapy. This is exemplified in Katherine's case:

Katherine: [My counsellor] helped me get rid of the deeprooted stuff, a lot of the crap I've been containing, like looking at my childhood and upbringing, my relationships with my mother with whom I've felt very let down . . . to sort it out and cope with it, what tied me to my mum, what I really felt about it. Once she'd done that – we'd done it.

Women's basic viewpoint on social change may also have tended towards individualized solutions. Given – as in Katherine's experience – that what women had gained from feminist therapy was such an improvement on their previous emotional state, it may also have been hard to think of greater improvements (Mathiesen 1974). However, women's accounts of the benefits of feminist therapy were not accompanied by recognition that ending conditions such as Katherine had experienced (see Katherine Chapter 2, page 31) required changes in ideology and social policy relating to women's role in child care and the need to agitate for this (David and New 1985). Instead, as reflected in women's comments to this effect, the proliferation of feminist therapy centres was endorsed as the solution to problems of women's emotional wellbeing.

The need for initiatives beyond feminist therapy

Preceding discussion leaves the following conundrum unresolved. Through the nature of the relationship that could be created in feminist therapy, women's emotional wellbeing genuinely seemed to benefit. But to what extent can feminist therapy be regarded as the solution to women's emotional problems, given that apart from the relatively unsubordinated experience it can provide, the general social conditions implicated in women's emotional wellbeing remain unchanged? Drawing on the evidence of women's accounts in our study suggests the answer. The benefit to women's wellbeing from feminist therapy was genuine enough. However, even greater benefits are achievable if and as the general social conditions implicated in undermining women's emotional wellbeing are tackled. This is not to deride the happiness radiating from women's accounts, but to open up the following comment made after feminist therapy – 'You see me restored, as far as I'm going to be' – to further possibilities.

Bringing this about requires feminist action beyond feminist therapy and work explicitly concerned with women's mental health, allied to action which uncovers and dissolves social inequality in all its forms running throughout society. This is clearly a vast task and, given counter-tendencies, there is no guarantee of effectiveness, but these are the sort of efforts required.

The degree of change required through a variety of initiatives beyond feminist therapy, if the constituent elements of gender subordination and other dimensions to inequality which affect women's emotional wellbeing are to be tackled, is illustrated from Annie's experience. Two problems which Annie highlighted in her account of what brought her to feminist therapy are discussed. First, her daughter's dependence on her to resolve the problems presented by the onset of Multiple Sclerosis (MS), and second, the disregard of Annie's interests in the reorganization at her work.

Annie's daughter had turned to her as the prime source of support, as she faced the onset of MS. *Annie:* 'She needed me for support, but there was an element in it to put it in simple terms, "Mother makes it better" – but of course Mother couldn't. Mother could only help her to accept it, which was extraordinarily difficult.' No attempt is being made to argue away the demands of the physical conditions Annie's daughter faced. However, in relation to the cruel social conditions which could accompany them, the work of disability-rights activists comes into play. Research on disability rights carried out by disability-rights activists has demonstrated that much suffering accompanying people's experience of physical impairment stems from the limitations imposed by disablist discrimination, that such discrimination is endemic and that it is only through action to dispel this, that such suffering will be abated (Begum 1990; Oliver 1990). Moreover, disability-rights activism itself has been at the forefront of moves to change such a situation, including the struggle for adequate material resources under the control of disabled people in order to underwrite their independence (Oliver 1983). Meanwhile, women disability-rights activists have demonstrated that gendered assumptions about disability have to be challenged, to enable the women concerned not to have an inferior existence to men (Morris 1991). Such work can be seen as helpful to Annie's daughter, but also to Annie in what she faced with her.

Turning to the disregard of Annie's interests as a main grade social worker during a reorganization: 'Ten years of effort . . . the accumulation of experience and so on . . . counted for nothing, that I could suddenly be dropped and told to do something for which I had no experience at all.' The increasing tendency for social work employees to be subject to bureaucratic controls in their employment has been under scrutiny for some time (Corrigan and Leonard 1978). More recently the tendency for women employees to occupy the lower ranks as opposed to managerial posts has been highlighted (Howe 1986). As a consequence, women's opportunity to control the nature of their employment conditions is comparatively circumscribed, as in Annie's case. However, this in turn, has been understood as part of a more general picture of women's comparatively inferior employment conditions, which both reflect and reinforce women's subordinate social position (Hanmer and Statham 1988: Ch. 8). Moreover, the need has been identified for a gamut of action in trades unions, party politics, education, child care provision, and international politics, allied with ideological changes, to begin to produce a situation where women at least enjoy an equivalent position to men in the labour force (Dominelli 1991).

Bringing about the type of changes under discussion is not in the gift of feminist or anti-discriminatory activism. Powerful counter-thrusts to such goals are currently in operation. In Britain, at the time of writing, the material resources essential to secure independent living for people with disabilities are being eroded through government cutbacks. Plans are afoot to cut long-term benefits (George 1993). Benefits in kind have also been cut back through reduced funding to Social Services Departments (Ivory 1992). While women's part-time employment remains one of the growth areas in employment, employment opportunities generally have been decimated (Blackburn 1991: Ch. 1). Measures specifically to enhance women's participation in the labour market in Britain, such as universal state-funded day care provision remain moribund (Moss 1991).

The picture presented by this account of the type of action required to tackle the underlying social conditions implicated in women's emotional wellbeing suggests the following: Treating feminist therapy as a partial solution to what undermines women's emotional wellbeing does make sense. However, to treat feminist therapy as *the* solution risks undermining women's emotional wellbeing. It obscures the possibility of even greater happiness being attainable and the need for women's energies to go into a range of activities beyond feminist therapy to secure this.

Conclusion

On the evidence of women's experience here, this study's answer to the question of how egalitarian are the outcomes of feminist therapy is heavily qualified. In being so, it differs from the viewpoint of feminist therapy's critics and proponents alike (see Chapter 1).

For women undergoing profound emotional distress feminist therapy can have a positive effect. This is to the extent – but only to the extent – that it provides a rare experience of relative freedom from their emotional needs and resources being treated as inferior. As this happens, the women concerned gain a greater and enduring sense of self-worth and consequently greater emotional wellbeing. However, the range of feminist therapy seems limited in terms of reaching women in different social circumstances. Its capacity to take account of the impact of different social inequalities also seems limited. Therefore, it can result in compounding existing inequalities.

Feminist therapy also tends not to engage with certain dimensions to emotional wellbeing such as the dominant behaviour of others in women's lives and the contribution of other feminist/anti-discriminatory initiatives.

The indications are that initiatives beyond feminist therapy, tackling gender subordination and a range of unequal social conditions are necessary to women enjoying a fuller experience of emotional wellbeing.

For all these reasons, feminist therapy should be seen as a partial solution to redressing the profound social inequalities implicated in women's emotional welfare.

six
Conclusions: the contribution of feminist therapy and counselling to promoting women's emotional wellbeing

Introduction

This book has explored women's experience of feminist therapy. In doing so it has focused on the limitations to analysing the nature of women's emotional wellbeing solely in terms of subordination through gender, and on the egalitarian nature of the outcomes of feminist therapy. Its main conclusion is that feminist therapy only redresses the undermining effects of social inequalities on women's emotional wellbeing to the extent that in practice it provides an experience of relative freedom from subordination.

The principal perspectives, forms of practice and organization which from the evidence of this study need to inform feminist therapy, if it is to contribute to a more equitable experience of women's emotional wellbeing, are set out below. They are a blend of existing features and further developments. They also point to the importance of analysis of feminist therapy being derived from the views and experience of women participants in their own right as well as from practitioners. This does not guarantee that 'the last word' on feminist therapy is then available, but it does make it possible to begin to understand what is promising about it and what its limitations are.

Perspectives on women's emotional wellbeing

Women's emotional wellbeing cannot simply be conceptualized in generic terms. Taking account of how differential experience among women both undermines women's wellbeing and provides opportunities for solidarity in securing it is essential to any analysis.

Women should not be typified as passive psychological victims. This fails to do justice to the active and creative nature of their behaviour. The evidence from this study is that women do seek relationships which offer the opportunity for self-expression and receiving affection and that where the power relations involved enable this to happen, these dimensions to women's persona blossom.

Women's capacity for dominating behaviour also emerged in our study, its expression both contributing to and relative to existing power relations. This dimension to women's behaviour needs to be acknowledged. Otherwise there is a risk of disregarding a potential source of oppressive behaviour and also of truncating attempts to clarify its origins.

Evidence from this study also adds to the mass of existing feminist work which has uncovered how personal relationships – previously identified as *the* arena in which emotional needs are met, tend instead to be riddled with dominance and subordination. Therefore, it makes sense to visualize them not as self-contained entities but as sensitive to the impact of prevailing social inequalities.

Despite the pervasive character of social inequalities, the fluid nature of their effects also becomes apparent from women's accounts. Otherwise apparently equitable relationships could be mediated by a further dimension to inequality, to women's detriment. Alternatively, readily identifiable social hierarchies could yield relationships conducive to women's wellbeing. This suggests that hierarchical social relations should be seen as in a constant state of flux and consequently their impact on women's emotional wellbeing as variable. This is as opposed to seeing them as rigid tendencies which result in women's welfare being influenced in a consistent way.

The practice of feminist therapy

As described by one participant, feminist therapy can offer 'self-validation and some healing' and this is of immense benefit to the women concerned. However, it cannot be assumed that feminist therapy promotes emotional wellbeing. The evidence from this study is also that the theory and practice of feminist therapy can sidestep or reinforce existing forms of inequality as well as challenging them. Its power to create a more egalitarian experience of emotional wellbeing is relative to the extent that it contributes to the experience of freedom from subordination. The pedigree of its theories or forms of practice or organization cannot guarantee this, and in fact, despite their time-honoured or apparently radical or therapeutic identity, they may subvert this process. What matters is how the assumptions, resources and efforts of both the practitioners and women participants actually coalesce. For example, women appeared to benefit from engaging in feminist therapy when this meant engaging in a relationship characterized by relative freedom of expression – and one where their own emotional needs were valued, as were their efforts to meet other people's. However, such opportunities tended to be open only to limited populations of women. Also, only certain aspects of women's experience of inequality tended to be taken into account. Therefore, extending the reach and range of feminist therapy so it meets the diverse requirements of women and more truly meets women's needs is of prime importance.

The organization of feminist therapy

The immediate and wider organizational backdrop to feminist therapy emerges as integral to the quality of its practice. In common with many other feminist initiatives feminist therapy also faces pulling off a tricky dual requirement – enhancing existing cooperative working strategies, while negotiating support from and within central and local state institutions. Thus, as other commentators have suggested, the egalitarian nature of the organization of feminist therapy largely remains to be constructed. In this way it reflects the continued impact and influence of existing social inequalities. Nevertheless, the indications from this study are that the welfare of both women participants and practitioners does benefit from the degree to which representative and cooperative administrative structures are created.

Wider practice to promote women's emotional wellbeing

Finally, this study suggests that the practice of feminist therapy at its best needs to be seen as providing only a partial solution to the problem of securing women's emotional wellbeing. If women's emotional wellbeing is to be promoted, it cannot be walled off as a separate 'emotional' state only amenable to 'therapeutic' intervention. Realizing women's emotional wellbeing requires a different, more complex and extensive range of initiatives in addition to feminist therapy – tackling the unequal nature of social relations beyond gender subordination alone.

This seems a daunting project and against the grain of current political tendencies. However, two positive conclusions can be drawn. First, once the practice necessary to achieve a more equitable experience of women's emotional wellbeing is conceptualized in a wider way, then the greater wealth of human resources already engaged in such practice becomes apparent. Second, progress on this wider project means women's emotional wellbeing should improve.

Appendix 1: sampling and interviewing procedures

Introduction

The main features of this study's design have been presented in Chapter 1. The empirical material on which the study is based derives from interviews with the counsellors, coordinator, and a sample of the population of women participants at a provincial feminist therapy centre across its first two years of operation. Here the nature of the sampling and interviewing procedures and the conditions under which they were carried out are described to clarify how this material was obtained.

The counsellors and coordinator

The counsellors and coordinator were keen to participate in the research as they felt that the credibility of feminist therapy was increased by being open to independent scrutiny. They also thought that the publication of such work would help to make the nature of feminist therapy more widely known. As a researcher, I met their criteria for access. These were that I was someone with direct experience of feminist practice, and therefore likely to appreciate its demands, and someone whose work they thought had demonstrated sensitivity to the emotional vicissitudes women faced.

Each counsellor was interviewed by me on four occasions. The series of four interviews each lasting about one-and-half hours were taped, later transcribed and rendered anonymous. They covered the following issues:

1 An account of the nature of the counsellor's involvement in the Centre, focusing on what they identified as the main aims, perspectives and

principles informing their own practice and that of the collective and its organization as a whole.

2 An account of their individual practice. This concentrated on the resources and varieties of method they employed and the outcomes as they perceived them for the women concerned and for themselves.

3 The counsellors' observations on the extent to which personal relationships which women participants identified as primary met their emotional needs in childhood and adulthood. In relation to these observations, the counsellors were invited to discuss what they perceived to be the influence of the gendered nature of social relations or of other social divisions.

4 The counsellors were interviewed on their observations relating to women's previous therapeutic experience, if any, and women's experience at the Centre. The counsellors' views were obtained on the reasons why women came, the outcomes of participation and the nature of their evidence for this.

The first and second interviews were conducted on the same basis with the coordinator, but with amendments as appropriate, e.g. she was invited to describe the resources she drew on in her work. Interviews three and four were not viewed as relevant, except for issues relating to why women came to the Centre, and the outcomes of the coordinator's work.

The interviews were semi-structured, i.e. based on schedules to facilitate coverage of what had been identified as certain key issues, but also aiming to provide the counsellors with ample opportunity to raise and discuss other issues they identified as significant (Graham 1983; Finch 1984).

In the course of interviewing, to protect confidentiality, all references to third parties other than current colleagues were anonymous.

The interviews were carried out across the summer–autumn of 1986, approximately two years after the Centre had come into being. The assumption was that this provided time for significant patterns of work and experience to have become apparent.

Women participants

Christina Hughes and I collaborated in carrying out the sampling and interviewing of women participants. Christina Hughes' previous research experience was seen as very appropriate to the current project. It concerned detailed qualitative analysis from a feminist perspective, of women's experience of a specific personal relationship – step-parenting (Hughes 1991).

Making contact

The two principal aims of interviewing were: first, to gain a picture of the significance for participants' emotional wellbeing of what they identified as primary personal relationships in childhood and adulthood; second, to gain their detailed accounts of the significance of feminist therapy for their emotional wellbeing.

We were fortunate enough to be advised on our aims and approach by two women currently participating in feminist therapy. One was White, the other South Asian. They suggested, as proved to be the case, that women coming to the Centre would be keen to share their experience, to help other women. They also thought – as again proved to be the case – that women participants would be prepared to be critical of the Centre's work, on the grounds that women participants would see this as benefiting other women. Our advisers' view was that our independent position and strict adherence to confidentiality would foster such a critical approach. As confidentiality was at a premium, given the nature of all the material under discussion in the interviews, they also advised us to check with the co-ordinator as to the best means of initial contact. For example, letters might not be appropriate.

As women participants wished, the interviews took place either at their houses, in interviewing rooms we had access to, or in the Centre. With the women's agreement, they were taped, transcribed later and rendered anonymous. The average interview was two hours, with breaks and/or follow-up, as met the women's individual requirements. They were conducted across the summer of 1987 to spring 1988.

Sampling

Within the resources of the study the main aim was to obtain evidence of women participants' experience of the outcomes of feminist therapy. This meant obtaining a cross-section of experience of the following: the main forms of intervention, i.e. one-to-one counselling, group work and initial assessment interviews; the different lengths of contact, and the work of all four counsellors.

Even if the numbers were small, it also meant interviewing women after feminist therapy ended. This provided the opportunity to probe how the outcomes of feminist therapy fared, once participants' contact with the Centre had ceased. Moreover, interviewing while feminist therapy was in progress might have made it difficult to deduce which shortcomings were due to unfinished business. This approach also had the further advantage of being in keeping with our view that it was not acceptable to interview women currently engaging in feminist therapy, as this input inadvertently interferes with its processes. Therefore, women were interviewed at least six months after their participation in feminist therapy had ended.

We did not sample to compensate for the under-representation of women in certain social circumstances in the work of the Centre, e.g. women from minority ethnic groups. Instead, we hypothesized that our sampling was likely to result in a profile of social circumstances amongst women participants similar to that represented in the Centre's work. Thus, as such it would reflect the nature of the Centre's actual constituency. This proved to be the case for the most part. For example, an evaluation of the Centre's first two years work, made available to us, revealed that only 5 per cent of participants were non-White; only 3 per cent (four) were aged over 60, with the median age of participants being 34 years old. The incidence of physical disability was not recorded. This compared with the following profile of the female population for the area the Centre served, which was obtained from statistics derived from Census returns: 21 per cent of women were non-White; 23 per cent of women were aged over 60. In our sample, 5 per cent (one) of the women were non-White. No woman was aged over 60, the oldest were in their mid-fifties, the median age was 33 years old. One woman was disabled.

An anonymous record was obtained from the counsellors of all the one-to-one counselling and group work they had carried out from the opening of the Centre, and which had ended six months previously. This yielded 21 cases of one-to-one counselling. This number was then reduced to 15 for interviewing. In two cases contact between the counsellor concerned and the women participants had ceased abruptly and no further address was available. In two other cases contact had been so infrequent and sporadic that we considered they were not viable as examples of continuous work. To even up the proportion of cases representing the work of different counsellors, we then further reduced at random by two the numbers from one counsellor's caseload.

Of fifteen women to be interviewed, one refused. In another case the tape was accidentally voided after the interview. In total, thirteen women who had had experience of one-to-one counselling across a period of three months to three years and representing examples of the work of all the counsellors were interviewed (see Appendix 2).

We also selected at random two members from each of two therapeutic groups (total group membership five and six respectively). These groups had been originally led by the counsellors, and then become self-help groups. All the women contacted agreed to be interviewed, but subsequently one woman became ill and it was impossible to pursue interviewing. Therefore, three women were interviewed (see Appendix 2).

Finally, all the women we interviewed had had experience of initial assessment interviews. Nevertheless, to complement this we wanted to gain some impression of women's views on whether such interviews were important pieces of work in their own right, as the counsellors had maintained. We also wanted to do so while the memory of such interviews might still be freshly in mind. The counsellors were each asked to nominate two initial assessment interviews across the past six months (total of such interviews: 32). They were asked to base their choice on interviews which they viewed as having a positive outcome, e.g. resolution of a problem, or referral. From this list we chose one woman at random per counsellor to contact, i.e. four in all. All the women concerned agreed to be interviewed, but then, despite repeated attempts, it proved impossible to contact one woman. This left three women in this category (see Appendix 2).

Interviewing

As with the counsellors' interviews, the interviews with women participants were semi-structured. They addressed the following issues. First, women were invited to identify what were the most important personal relationships to them in childhood and adulthood. Second, they were asked to describe the positive and negative effects of these relationships on their emotional wellbeing. Third, they were asked to describe the reasons they went to the Centre, the nature and effects of intervention at the time, their experience of contact ceasing, the subsequent effects if any, of engaging in feminist therapy, and any criticisms of the work.

Analysing the data

After interviewing was completed, work on analysing the data was suspended for 18 months as a result of my lengthy recovery from a viral illness. The data produced from interviews with the counsellors, the coordinator and the women participants was then analysed until clear themes relating to the original lines of enquiry emerged. These themes were then subjected again to challenge against the data and further refined to produce the basis of the arguments, with supporting evidence, used in this study.

Appendix 2: profile of the sample of women participants

Pseudonym	Age	Ethnic identity	Identified self as disabled as a result of a physical impairment; or as having serious health problems	Occupation
Annie	Mid-50s	White British	Serious physical health problems	Social work
Beatrice	Early 40s	White British	Serious physical health problems	Secretary
Christine	Early 30s	White British		Social work
Debbie	Early 30s	White British		Home care
Esther	Mid-40s	White British		Teaching
Frances	Early 30s	White British		Media
Gillian	Early 20s	African-Caribbean British born		Secretary
Irene	Mid-20s	White British	Disabled	Social work
Jan	Early 30s	White British		Community work
Katherine	Mid-30s	White British		Social work
Louise	Mid-50s	White British	Serious physical health problems	Theatre
Mary	Late 30s	White British		Further education
Nina	Early 40s	White Continental European		Further education
Olivia	Early 30s	White British		Teaching
Ruth	Late 30s	White British		Lecturing – currently unemployed
Sue	Late 30s	White British		Civil service
Tina	Mid-20s	White British		Student
Winifred	Early 50s	White British		Teacher
Zoë	Early 30s	White British		Computing

Current partners	Children	Previous treatment/ therapy/ counselling	Nature of contact with Centre Counsellor	Identity of Counsellor involved. To protect confidentiality, different identities have been indicated by a, b, c, d.
Male	Yes	No	1 to 1 counselling 12 months	b
Male	No	No	1 to 1 counselling 4 months	b
Male	Yes	Yes	1 to 1 counselling 2 years	c
Male	Yes	Yes	1 to 1 counselling 7 months	b
Male Female	Yes	Yes	1 to 1 counselling 19 months	d
Male	No	Yes	1 to 1 counselling 21 months	a
Male	Yes	Yes	1 to 1 counselling 3 months	d
Male	No	Yes	Groupwork	c/d
Female	No	No	1 to 1 counselling 9 months	d
Male	Yes	No	1 to 1 counselling 18 months	c
Male	Yes	No	Assessment interview	b
Male	Yes	No	1 to 1 counselling 4 months	c
Female	Yes	No	1 to 1 counselling 19 months	a
Male	No	Yes	Assessment interview	a
Male Female	No	Yes	Groupwork	c/d
Male	No	No	Assessment interview	c
Female	No	No	Groupwork	a/b
Male	Yes	Yes	1 to 1 counselling 3 years	b
Male	No	Yes	1 to 1 counselling 2 years	a

Appendix 3: profile of the counsellors and coordinator at the centre

Counsellors – pseudonyms:

Elspeth
Fran
Miriam
Rosemary

Coordinator pseudonym:
Bridget

Identity

To help preserve confidentiality (by making it more difficult to identify women in the sample engaging in feminist therapy, through the identity of the counsellor) the following features of the counsellors' and coordinator's identity are described collectively.

All were White British, currently had male partners, and with one exception had children. Their ages ranged from late 30s to early 60s with the majority in their late 30s. One identified herself as having a physical impairment.

Note All references to third parties on the part of women participants and counsellors are also rendered in pseudonyms.

References

Ahmed, S. (1986) Cultural racism in work with Asian women and girls. In Ahmed, S., Cheetham, J. and Small, J. (eds) *Social Work with Black Children and Their Families*. London, Batsford.

Aldridge, J. and Becker, S. (1993) *Children Who Care*. Loughborough, Department of Social Sciences, Loughborough University.

Andrews, B. (1989) A kind of loving, *The Guardian*, 23 May.

Ardill, S. and O'Sullivan, S. (1986) Upsetting an applecart: difference, desire and lesbian sadomasochism, *Feminist Review*, 23, 31–58.

Bain, O. and Sanders, M. (1990) *Out in the Open*. London, Virago Upstarts.

Baker Miller, J. (1978) *Toward a New Psychology of Women*. Harmondsworth, Penguin.

Barnes, M. and Maple, N. (1992) *Women and Mental Health: Challenging the Stereotypes*. Birmingham, Venture Press.

Barrett, M. and McIntosh, M. (1982) *The Anti-social Family*. London, Verso.

Begum, N. (1990) *The Burden of Gratitude*. Coventry, Department of Applied Social Studies, University of Warwick and Social Care Association.

Berne, E. (1961) *Transactional Analysis in Psychotherapy*. New York, Grove Press.

Berne, E. (1968) *Games People Play*. Harmondsworth, Penguin.

Binney, V., Harkell, G. and Nixon, J. (1981) *Leaving Violent Men: A Study of Refugees and Housing for Battered Women*. Leeds, Womens Aid Federation.

Blackburn, C. (1991) *Poverty and Health: Working with Families*. Milton Keynes, Open University Press.

Blaxter, M. (1990) *Health and Lifestyles*. London, Tavistock/Routledge.

Broverman, I., Broverman, D., Clarkson, F. et al. (1970) Sex role stereotypes and clinical judgements of mental health, *Journal of Consulting and Clinical Psychology*, 34(1), 1–7.

Brown, G.W., Andrews, B., Harris, T. et al. (1986) Social support self esteem and depression, *Psychological Medicine*, 16, 813–31.

Brown, L. (1990) The meaning of a multicultural perspective for theory building in feminist therapy, *Women and Therapy*, Special Edition, 9(112), 1–21.

Brown, L. (1992) While waiting for the revolution: the case for a lesbian feminist psychotherapy, *Feminism and Psychology*, 2(2), 239–53.

Brown, L.S. and Liss-Levinson, N. (1981) Feminist therapy I. In Corsini, R.J. (ed.) *Handbook of Innovative Psychotherapies*. New York, Wiley-Interscience.

Bryan, B. and Dadzie, S. (1985) *The Heart of the Race*. London, Virago.

Burstow, B. (1992) *Radical Feminist Therapy – Working in the Context of Violence*. Newbury Park, California, Sage.

Busfield, J. (1989) Sexism and psychiatry, *Sociology*, 23(3), 343–64.

Butler, S. and Wintram, C. (1991) *Feminist Groupwork*. London, Sage.

Calvert, J. (1985) Motherhood. In Brook, E. and Davis, A. (eds) *Women, The Family and Social Work*. London, Tavistock.

Cervi, B. (1993) Divorce cases highlight Children Act loopholes, *Community Care*, 956, 4 March.

Chaplin, J. (1988) *Feminist Counselling in Action*. London, Sage.

Chernin, K. (1985) *The Hungry Self: Women, eating and identity*. New York, Times Books.

Chesler, P. (1972) *Women and Madness*. New York, Doubleday.

Cohen, G. (1978) Women's solidarity and the preservation of privilege. In Caplan, P. and Bujra, J. (eds) *Women United, Women Divided*. London, Tavistock.

Commission for Racial Equality (1993) *The Sorrow in my Heart – Sixteen Asian Women Speak About Depression*. London, Commission for Racial Equality.

Conway, J. (ed.) (1988) *Prescription for Poor Health – the Crisis for Homeless Families*. London, London Food Commission, Maternity Alliance, SHAC, Shelter.

Corrigan, P. and Leonard, P. (1978) *Social Work Under Capitalism*. London, Macmillan.

Crawford, J., Kippax, S., Onyx, J. et al. (1992) *Emotion and Gender – Constructing Meaning from Memory*. London, Sage.

Cross, M. (1984) Feminism and the disability movement. In Holland, J. (ed.) *Feminist Action I*. London, Battle Axe Books.

Curno, A., Lamming, A., Leach, L., et al. (1982) *Women in Collective Action*. London, The Association of Community Workers.

David, M. and New, C. (1985) *For the Children's Sake: Making Childcare More Than Women's Business*. Harmondsworth, Penguin.

Dobash, R.E. and Dobash, R. (1980) *Violence Against Wives: A Case Against the Patriarchy*. London, Open Books.

Dobash, R.E. and Dobash, R.P. (1992) *Women, Violence and Social Change*. London, Routledge.

Dominelli, L. (1988) *Anti-racist Social Work*. London, Macmillan.

Dominelli, L. (1991) *Women Across Continents*. Hemel Hempstead, Harvester Wheatsheaf.

Dominelli, L. and McLeod, E. (1989) *Feminist Social Work*. London, Macmillan.

Donnelly, A. (1986) *Feminist Social Work with a Woman's Group*. Monograph 41, Norwich, University of East Anglia.

Dworkin, S. (1984) Traditionally defined client meet feminist therapist: feminist therapy as attitude changes, *The Personal Guidance Journal*, Jan 1984, 301–5.

Egan, G. (1975) *The Skilled Helper*. Monterey, California, Brooks/Cole.

Eichenbaum, L. and Orbach, S. (1982) *Outside in, Inside Out. Women's Psychology: A Feminist Psychoanalytic Approach.* Harmondsworth, Penguin.

Eichenbaum, L. and Orbach, S. (1984) *What do Women Want?* London, Fontana.

Eichenbaum, L. and Orbach, S. (1985) *Understanding Women.* London, Penguin.

Eichenbaum, L. and Orbach, S. (1987) Separation and intimacy: crucial practice issues in working with women in therapy. In Ernst, S. and Maguire, M. (eds) *Living with the Sphinx – Papers from the Women's Therapy Centre.* London, The Women's Press.

Eichenbaum, L. and Orbach, S. (1988) *Bittersweet, Facing up to Feelings of Love, Envy and Competition in Women's Friendships.* London, Arrow Books.

Elliott, M. (ed.) (1993) *Female Sexual Abuse of Children – the Ultimate Taboo.* High Harlow, Essex, Longman.

Ernst, S. and Goodison, L. (1981) *In Our Own Hands: A Book of Self-help Therapy.* London, The Women's Press.

Ernst, S. and Maguire, M. (eds) (1987) *Living with the Sphinx – Papers from the Women's Therapy Centre.* London, The Women's Press.

Fairbairn, W.R.D. (1952) *Psychoanalytic Studies of the Personality.* London, Tavistock.

Finch, J. (1984) It's great to have someone to talk to: the ethics and politics of interviewing women. In Bell, C. and Roberts, H. (eds). *Social Researching: Politics, Problems and Practice.* London, Routledge and Kegan Paul.

Forisba, B.L. (1981) Feminist therapy. In Corsini, R. (ed.) *Handbook of Innovative Therapies.* New York, Wiley.

Fox Harding, L. (1991) *Perspectives in Child Care Policy.* London, Longman.

Freud, S. (1973) *An Outline of Psychoanalysis.* London, The Hogarth Press. (Originally published 1940)

Frost, N. (1992) Implementing the Children Act 1989 in a hostile climate. In Carter, P., Jeffs, T. and Smith, M.K. (eds) *Changing Social Work and Welfare.* Milton Keynes, Open University Press.

Gelb, J. (1990) Feminism in Britain: Politics without power. In Dahlerup, D. (ed.) *The New Women's Movement – Feminism and Political Power in Europe and the USA.* London, Sage.

George, M. (1993) Cause and effect, *Community Care,* 15 July, Issue No. 975, 22–3.

Gilbert, L.A. (1980) Feminist therapy. In Brodsky, A.M. and Hare-Mustin, R.T. (eds) *Women and Psychotherapy – An Assessment of Research and Practice.* New York, The Guilford Press.

Gorman, J. (1992) *Out of the Shadows.* London, MIND Publications.

Graham, H. (1983) Do her answers fit his questions? Women and the survey method. In Gamarnika, E., Morgan, D., Purvis, J. et al. (eds) *The Public and Private.* London, Heinemann.

Graham, H. (1984) *Women, Health and the Family.* Hemel Hempstead, Harvester Wheatsheaf.

Graham, H. (1992) Feminism and social work education. *Issues in Social Work Education,* 11(2), 48–64.

Graham, H. (1993) *Hardship and Health in Women's Lives.* Hemel Hempstead, Harvester Wheatsheaf.

Guntrip, H. (1968) *Schizoid Phenomena, Object Relations and the Self*. London, Hogarth.

Hamblin, A. (1983) Is a feminist heterosexuality possible? In Cartledge, S. and Ryan, I. (eds) *Sex and Hope. New Thoughts on Old Contradictions*. London, The Women's Press.

Hanmer, J. and Statham, D. (1988) *Women and Social Work: Towards A Woman-Centred Practice*. London, Macmillan.

Heenan, M.C. (1988) A two-part study to establish the values held by feminist therapists with a view to examining whether these are communicated to their clients in sessions. Unpublished M.Sc. in Psychotherapy. Coventry, Department of Psychology, University of Warwick.

Hemmings, S. (1982) *Girls are Powerful*. London, Sheba.

Hemmings, S. (1985) *A Wealth of Experience*. London, Pandora Press.

Hite, S. (1987) *Women and Love: A Cultural Revolution in Progress*. New York, Knopf.

Hochschild, A. (1990) *The Second Shift: Working Parents and the Revolution at Home*. London, Piatkus.

Holland, S. (1989) 'Women and community mental health – twenty years on', *Clinical Psychology Forum*, 22: 35–7.

Holland, S. (1990) Psychotherapy, oppression and social action: gender, race, and class in black women's depression. In Perelberg, R.J. and Miller, A. (eds) *Gender and Power in Families*. London, Tavistock/Routledge.

Holland, S. (1992) From social abuse to social action – a neighbourhood psychotherapy and social action project for women. In Ussher, J.M. and Nicolson, P. (eds) *Gender Issues in Clinical Psychology*. London, Routledge.

Howe, D. (1986) The segregation of women and their work in the personal social services. In *Critical Social Policy*, 15, Spring, 21–36.

Hudson, A. (1989) Changing perspectives: feminism, gender and social work. In Langan, M. and Lee, P. (eds) *Radical Social Work Today*. London, Unwin Hyman.

Hudson, A. (1992) The child sexual abuse 'industry' and gender relations in social work. In Langan, M. and Day, L. (eds) *Women, Oppression and Social Work Issues in Anti-Discriminatory Practice*. London, Routledge.

Hughes, B. and Mtezuka, M. (1992) Social work and older women: where have older women gone? In Langan, M. and Day, L. (eds) *Women, Oppression and Social Work Issues in Anti-Discriminatory Practice*. London, Routledge.

Hughes, C. (1991) *Stepparents: Wicked or Wonderful?* Aldershot, Avebury.

Ivory, M. (1992) Funding announcement heralds major cuts, *Community Care*, 3 December 1992, 1.

Jackins, H. (1978) *The Upward Trend*. Seattle, Rational Island Publishers.

Jacobs, M. (1984) Psychodynamic therapy: the Freudian Approach. In Dryden, W. (ed.) *Individual Therapy in Britain*. London, Harper and Row.

Johnson, J.L. (1991) Learning to live again: the process of adjustment following a heart attack. In Morse, J.M. and Johnson, J.L. (eds) *The Illness Experience, Dimensions of Suffering*. Newbury Park, California, Sage.

Kareem, J. and Littlewood, R. (1992) *Intercultural Therapy, Themes, Interpretations and Practice*. Oxford, Blackwell Scientific Publications.

Kelly, L. (1988) *Surviving Sexual Violence*. Cambridge, Polity.

Kelly, L. (1991) Unspeakable acts: women who abuse, *Trouble and Strife*, Summer 91, 13–21.

Kitzinger, S. (1985) *Woman's Experience of Sex*. Harmondsworth, Penguin.

Knowles, J.P. and Cole, E. (1990) *Woman-defined Motherhood*. New York, Harrington Park Press.

Langan, M. (1992) Introduction: women and social work in the 1990s. In Langan, M. and Day, L. (eds) *Women, Oppression and Social Work*. London, Routledge.

Langan, M. and Day, L. (1992) *Women, Oppression and Social Work – Issues in Anti-discriminatory Practice*. London, Routledge.

Lawrence, M. (1984) *The Anorexic Experience*. London, The Women's Press.

Laws, S. (1991) Women on the verge: Brixton Women's Counselling Service, *Trouble and Strife*, 20, 8–12.

Leonard, P. and McLeod, E. (1980) *Marital Violence: Social Construction and Social Service Response*. Coventry, Department of Applied Social Studies, University of Warwick.

Lobel, K. (ed.) (1986) *Naming the Violence: Speaking Out About Lesbian Battering*. Seattle, Seal Press.

Louisa Lawson Centre (1992) *The Louisa Lawson Centre Annual Report*. Available from 112 West Botany Street, Arncliffe, New South Wales, 2205, Australia, The Louisa Lawson Centre for Counselling and Therapy for Women.

Macdonald, B. and Rich, C. (1984) *Look Me in the Eye*. London, The Women's Press.

Maguire, M. (1987) Casting the evil eye – women and envy. In Ernst, S. and Maguire, M. (eds) *Living with the Sphinx – Papers from the Women's Therapy Centre*. London, The Women's Press.

Mama, A. (1989) *The Hidden Struggle: Statutory and Voluntary Sector Responses to Violence Against Black Women in the Home*. London, London Race and Housing Research Unit.

Mathiesen, T. (1974) *The Politics of Abolition*. Oxford, Martin Robertson.

McLeod, E. (1982) *Women Working: Prostitution Now*. London, Croom Helm.

Mearns, D. and Dryden, W. (1990) *Experiences of Counselling in Action*. London, Sage.

Metcalf, A. and Humphries, M. (eds) (1985) *The Sexuality of Men*. London, Pluto Press.

Mihill, C. (1993) Plea to eject psychologist sex abusers, *The Guardian*, 5 April.

Miles, A. (1988) *Women and Mental Illness*. Brighton, Harvester Wheatsheaf.

Miller, A. (1988) *For Your Own Good, the Roots of Violence in Child Rearing*. London, Virago.

Miller, A. (1989) *The Drama of Being a Child*. London, Virago.

Morgan, D.H.J. (1992) *Discovering Men*. London, Routledge.

Morris, J. (1991) *Pride Against Prejudice: Transforming Attitudes to Disability*. London, The Women's Press.

Moss, P. (1991) Day care for young children in the United Kingdom. In Melhuish, E.C. and Moss, P. (eds) *Day Care for Young Children: International Perspectives*. London, Routledge.

Nelson-Jones, R. (1988) *Practical Counselling and Helping Skills*. London, Cassell.

Newall, P. (1989) *Children are People Too: The Case Against Corporal Punishment*. London, Bedford Press.

Newson, J. and Newson, E. (1976) Day-to-day aggression between parent and child. In Tutt, N. (ed.) *Violence*. London, DHSS, HMSO.

Norwood, R. (1986) *Women Who Love Too Much*. London, Arrow Books.

Norwood, R. (1988) *Letters from Women who Love too Much, a Closer Look at Relationship Addiction and Recovery*. London, Arrow Books.

Oakley, A. (1976) *Housewife*. Harmondsworth, Penguin Books.

O'Connor, P. (1992) *Friendships Between Women – A Critical Review*. Hemel Hempstead, Harvester Wheatsheaf.

Oldfield, S. (1983) *The Counselling Relationship – A Study of the Client's Experience*. London, Routledge and Kegan Paul.

Oliker, S.J. (1989) *Best Friends and Marriage: Exchange Among Women*. California, University of California Press.

Oliver, M. (1983) *Social Work with Disabled People*. London, Macmillan.

Oliver, M. (1990) *The Politics of Disablement*. Basingstoke, Macmillan.

OPCS (1990) *Morbidity Statistics from General Practice, 1981–82: Socio-economic Analysis*. OPCS Series MB5 (1), London, HMSO.

Pahl, J. (1985) *Private Violence and Public Policy*, London, Routledge, Kegan Paul.

Payne, S. (1991) *Women Health and Poverty*. Hemel Hempstead, Harvester Wheatsheaf.

Penfold, S. and Walker, G. (1984) *Women and the Psychiatric Paradox*. Milton Keynes, Open University Press.

Perkins, R. (1991) Therapy for lesbians? The case against? *Feminism and Psychology*, 1(3), 325–38.

Perls, F.S. (1969) *Gestalt Therapy Verbatim*. Lafayette, Real People Press.

Perls, F.C. (1976) *The Gestalt Approach and Eye Witness to Therapy*. Des Plaines, Bantam Books.

Phillips, A. and Rakusen, J. (1989) *The New Bodies, Ourselves*. Harmondsworth, Penguin.

Phoenix, A. (1991) *Young Mothers?* London, Polity Press.

Pitkeathly, J. (1989) *It's My Duty Isn't It? The Plight of Carers in Our Society*. London, Souvenir Press.

Popay, J. (1992) My health is all right, but I'm just tired all the time. Women's experience of ill health. In Roberts, H. (ed.) *Women's Health Matters*. London, Routledge.

Quick, A. and Wilkinson, R. (1991) *Income and Health*. London, Socialist Health Association.

Ramazanoglou, C. (1989) *Feminism and the Contradictions of Oppression*. London, Routledge.

Raymond, J. (1986) *A Passion for Friends*. London, The Women's Press.

Reid, W.T. and Epstein, L. (1977) *Task Centred Practice*. New York, Columbia University Press.

Roberts, H. (1985) *The Patient Patients, Women and their Doctors*. London, Pandora Press.

Rogers, C.R. (1961) *On Becoming A Person*. Boston, Houghton Mifflin.

Rosewater, L.B. and Walker, L.E. (1985) Introduction – feminist therapy: a coming of age. In Rosewater, L.B. and Walker, L.W. (eds) *Handbook of Feminist Therapy: Women's Issues in Psychotherapy*. New York, Springer.

Rowbotham, S. (1989) *The Past is Before Us, Feminism in Action Since the 1960s*. London, Penguin Books.

Rowland, R. (1993) Radical feminist heterosexuality: the personal and the political. In Wilkinson, S. and Kitzinger, C. (eds) *Heterosexuality*. London, Sage.

Rubin, L.B. (1985) *Just Friends: The Role of Friendships in Our Lives*. New York, Harper Row.

Ryan, B. and Stubbs, P. (1989) Child centered practice in sexual abuse, *Practice*, Autumn/Winter 3 and 4, 222–34.

Ryan, J. (1983) *Feminism and Therapy: Pam Smith Memorial Lecture*. London, Polytechnic of North London.

Sarsby, J. (1983) *Romantic Love and Society*. Harmondsworth, Penguin.

Sayers, J. (1988) My mother, my therapist, *Women's Review of Books*, 5(70), 22.

Seidler, V. (1991) *The Achilles' Heel Reader*. London, Routledge.

Shah, N. (1989) It's up to you sisters: black women and radical social work. In Langan, M. and Lee, P. (eds) *Radical Social Work Today*. London, Unwin Hyman.

Smith, A. and Jacobson, B. (1989) *The Nation's Health – A Strategy for the 1990s*. London, The Kings Fund.

Spackman, A. (1991) *The Health of Informal Carers*. Southampton, Institute for Health Policy Studies, Southampton University.

Spring, J. (1987) *Cry Hard and Swim*. London, Virago.

Stacey, M. and Price, M. (1981) *Women Power and Politics*. Tavistock, London.

Sturdivant, S. (1980) *Therapy with Women: A Feminist Philosophy of Treatment*. New York, Springer.

Sturdy, C. (1987) Questioning the Sphinx: an experience of working in a women's organisation. In Ernst, S. and Maguire, M. (eds) *Living with the Sphinx – Papers from the Women's Therapy Centre*. London, The Women's Press.

Swain, S.O. (1992) Men's friendships with women – intimacy, sexual boundaries and the informant role. In Nardi, P.M. (ed.) *Men's Friendships*. Newbury Park, California, Sage.

Thorne, B. (1984) Person-Centred Therapy. In Dryden, W., *Individual Therapy in Britain*. London, Harper and Row.

Truax, C.B. and Carkhuff, R.R. (1975) *Towards Effective Counselling and Psychotherapy*. Chicago, Aldine.

Turkel, A.R. (1976) The impact of feminism on the practice of a woman analyst, *American Journal of Psychoanalysis*, 36, 119–26.

Ussher, J.M. (1991) *Women's madness: misogyny or mental illness*. Hemel Hempstead, Harvester Wheatsheaf.

Valentine, M. (1989) Developing a critical theory of child abuse: a discussion of the nature of child abuse as a manifestation of the social order. Unpublished PhD Thesis, Coventry, Department of Applied Social Studies, University of Warwick.

Walker, M. (1990) *Women in Therapy and Counselling*. Milton Keynes, Open University Press.

Wallbank, S. (1992) The secret world of bereaved children. In Varma, V.P. (ed.) *The Secret Life of Vulnerable Children*. London, Routledge.

Ward, E. (1984) *Father–Daughter Rape*. London, The Women's Press.

Watson, G. and Williams, J. (1992) Feminist practice in therapy. In Ussher, J.M. and Nicolson, P. (eds) *Gender Issues in Clinical Psychology*. Routledge, London.

Weedon, C. (1987) *Feminist Practice and Poststructural Theory*. Oxford, Basil Blackwell.

Wellington Eating Disorder Support (1992) *EDS – Wellington Eating Disorder Support*. Available from PO Box 5128, Lambton Quay, Wellington, New Zealand, Wellington Eating Disorder Support.

Wilkinson, S. and Kitzinger, C. (eds) (1993) *Heterosexuality*. London, Sage.

Williams, C.T. (1992) Women with learning difficulties are women too. In Langan, M. and Day, L. (eds) *Women Oppression and Social Work*. London, Routledge.

Willmott, P. (1987) *Friendship Networks and Social Support*. London, Policy Studies Institute.

Wing, J.K. and Bebbington, (1982) Epidemiology of depressive disorders in the community, *Journal of Affective Disorders*, 4, 331–45.

Winnicott, D.W. (1975) *Through Paediatrics to Psychoanalysis*. London, Tavistock.

Witherspoon, S. and Prior, S. (1991) Working mothers: free to choose. In Jowell, R., Brook, L. and Taylor, B. (eds) *British Social Attitudes: The 8th Report*. Aldershot, Dartmonth Publishing Co.

Women in Mind (1986) *Finding Our Own Solutions: Women's Experience of Mental Health Care*. London, MIND.

Woodward, J. (1988) *Understanding Ourselves*. London, Macmillan.

Ylö, K. and Bograd, M. (1988) *Feminist Perspectives on Wife Abuse*. Newbury Park, California, Sage.

Index

males, *see* men
marginalization, of women's different
      experience, 133–5
marriage, 57, 58, 70
   and female friendships, 77
   older women's accounts of, 13
maternal-infant relations, 19
medical practitioners, and sexism, 9
medical treatment of participants,
      117–18
memories, recalled through feminist
      therapy, 48–9
men
   anti-sexist writings of, 62
   effects of behaviour on women, 5
   and feminist therapy, 85, 87, 137–8
   friendships with, 56, 75, 76
   male partners
      of counsellors, 106, 107
      and the erosion of emotional
         wellbeing, 12–13
      sexist behaviour of, 59–61
      supportive behaviour of, 56, 61–3
   as medical practitioners, 9, 115
   relationships with, 56, 57–65
   as therapists, 18, 84
   women addicted to loving, 59
   and women's dominating behaviour,
      63–5
mother–daughter relationships
   in adulthood, 71
   in childhood, 10, 28–33, 52–3, 55
      and father's–mother's relationship,
         37–8
      and powerlessness of children,
         41–3, 45–6
   and counsellors as 'emotional
      midwives', 99–101
   and disabilities, 40, 50–1, 140
   sexist assumptions in, 82–3
   women's relationship with own
      children, 71–3
mothers
   of children with learning difficulties,
      8, 59–60
   parenting in poverty, 7–8, 13, 25,
      38–9
   relationships with, 10
   teenage, 39–40

National Health Service (NHS), 20,
      109–10

negative frames of reference,
      confronting and revising, 124–5
New Zealand, 1
non-directive counselling, 91–2
non-hierarchical counselling, 92–102

older women, 8, 20, 121
   accounts of marriage, 13
   marginalization of, 133
   and sexual relationships, 65
one-to-one counselling, 20, 23, 98, 123,
      137, 138

parents
   and the psychotherapeutic approach,
      88, 89–90
   relationships with in adulthood, 70–1
   see also fathers, relationships with;
      mother–daughter relationships
participants
   access to counselling, 120–1
   as active agents, 118
   criticisms of feminist therapy, 131–6
   emotional needs of, 122–3, 127–31
   and the enduring effects of feminist
      therapy, 130–1
   equality between counsellor and,
      18–19, 22
   experience of feminist therapy,
      112–42
   impact of social inequality, 113–15
   limitations of other sources of help,
      116–18
   medical treatment, 117–18
   and the organization of the Centre,
      102–5
   reasons for seeking feminist therapy,
      112–21
   relations with counsellors, 92–102
   rights, 19
   self-referral by, 95, 118, 120
   sense of being cared for, 123–4
   strengths, 19, 93–4
   in substantial distress, 112–13
passivity, self-denying, 79
pay, of counsellors, 106
person-centred/humanistic counselling,
      19–20, 21, 129
phobias, 114
physical disabilities, *see* disabilities
physical health, *see* health